"What a great role-model Rosy is for all who know her story! What a gift she has given her children… a mom with more energy to work and play, a mom who sets goals and achieves them, and a mom who is educated on healthful foods which are so important to growing bodies and brains. As a teacher, it is disheartening when I see so many T.V. commercials promoting treats, and so many unhealthy lunches coming to school. It is also interesting to note that students who come to school with goal-setting strategies and a "can-do" attitude are more motivated to work hard and are more likely to succeed in achieving their goals. I am sure that Rosy's spirited example of "taking charge" of her lifestyle, exchanging unhealthy habits for a healthier, life-affirming regimen of exercise and nutritious food will inspire many to set their sights on a worthy goal and work for it, as she did. Way to go, Rosy!"

Cathy Wilcox
Elementary School Teacher

I0438756

"Regular physical activity and healthy food choices are key factors in staying or becoming healthy. Rosy has demonstrated, that by surrounding one's self with the right support systems, investing the necessary time and energy and being committed to a personal wellness program, reaching one's goal is possible. We are pleased that the National Capital Region YMCA-YWCA has been part of Rosy's journey and we would like to congratulate Rosy on her successes!"

Kelly Shaw-Swettenham
National Capital Region YMCA-YWCA

*"This book will change your life!
Read it, absorb it, and take action! Say goodbye to failure.
Rosy will inspire you to get to the end without giving up."*

*Jean-Luc Boissonneault
Chelsea Boissonneault*

Authors of Abs on the Go
Owners of Free Form Fitness

"Here's what you'll get with Rosy: A real person with a real life, with everyday challenges, who's done something each of us with extra weight has wanted to do. Finally, once and for all, win the battle against the bulge."

Don Ermen
Assistant Managing Editor
Ottawa Sun

"The transformation that Rosy has made during the past year is truly the result of a sculptor at work. When one looks at her before she began the challenging workouts of the past year, one sees that it took not only a determined and dedicated individual, but one who challenged herself. To see her at the end of her year's journey, amazes me. I have been in the medical profession for more than forty years. I have witnessed many persons make huge successes in weight loss programs, but nothing like Rosy. She lost a whole person and has sculptured a body that truly is model quality. Presently, I serve as a member of the staff of Tony Little, the WORLD FAMOUS EXERCISE GURU. I handle the 'Before and After Success Story Program' for his organization, and was not only happy when Rosy made me aware of her SUCCESS STORY, I was happy as well that the equipment had been supplied by Tony's company, Health International Corporation, and had played a large part in her weight loss. I am personally very proud of you and your success story which I was honored to place on the Tony Little web site at www.tonylittle.com. Keep up the good work, Rosy, and please keep me apprised of your future healthy life success story. The BEST to YOU!"

Dr. Lloyd J. Minter
"Before and After Success Story Program"
Tony Little

"Rosy and Rob are a real testament to what willpower can do for your health. Their weight loss challenge began with one goal in mind and lots of ambition. The result: an inspiring transformation inside and out. Truly motivating! Way to go, girl!"

Erin Lannan
Producer
Rogers 22 "Daytime" Show

Rosy Moio Ghannai

breakin' free

How one woman defeated obesity in 12 months
and how you can too

Crowe Creations

Ottawa Canada

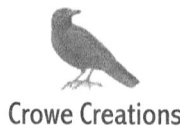

Crowe Creations

Ottawa Canada
crowecreations.ca
Info@crowecreations.ca

crowecreations.ca

First **Crowe Creations** Edition January 2009
Second Crowe Creations Edition January 2014

Designed by Crowe Creations

Text set in Book Antiqua; headings set in Bodoni MT Poster Compressed & Arial Narrow.

Cover design copyright © 2013 by Crowe Creations.

Photographs copyright © 2007, 2008 by Rosy Moio Ghannai & Chokri Ghannai; other photographs copyright © 2008 by Rosy Moio Ghannai & Gordon Chan.

ISBN: 978-0-9811737-0-2

CreateSpace
ISBN 13: 978-1494847753
ISBN 10: 1494847752

To my dad, Antonio Moio, the strongest man I know.

Acknowledgements

I would like to take a moment to thank editor and designer, Sherrill Wark of Crowe Creations, our publisher, for doing such an amazing job; Moe at Bradda Printing Services for the wonderful first edition; Free Form Fitness, Kanata; the YMCA-YWCA, Carlingwood; and my long-time friend and advisor, Christopher Quinton, of Sun Life Financial.

Thanks go to the media personnel who, to help inspire others, followed our story from the beginning: the *Ottawa Sun* newspaper; Rogers 22 "Daytime" show; and "iReport for CNN."

To all our friends from our Facebook group, and our blog, who have been there supporting our story from the beginning, it meant so much to us.

 Thanks to my entire family: Mom, Dad, Peter, Franca, Laura, Julia, Carla, Joel, nephews and nieces, for encouraging me to keep going even when times were tough. Couldn't have done it without you guys!

"We might not have much, but we have each other, and that makes us the RICHEST family in the world." — Antonio Moio ("Dad")

Special thanks to my husband, Chokri —a most patient man — for giving me the time I needed, which allowed me to do what I had to do throughout this process. I love and thank you! My wonderful kids, whom I love so dearly, Elisa, Adamo, and Emma: I did all this for you, so we could live the life we should have been living.

To my trainer, Robert "Scruff" Lagana: You have been my strength and mentor throughout this whole transformation. You have given me the proper tools to not only come out a winner, but to have the freedom, now, to live the way we ALL so richly deserve. Being obese took that away from me for most of my years. I could not have done this without you. Thanks for believing in me, and I will always be grateful. (hugz)

Thanks to you all!

Foreword

If there is, or ever was something that has held you back from being the best person you can be, this book is for you. It's a true-life, inspirational story about how one woman (me) came face to face with something that, for most of her years, had held her back: Obesity.

Obesity affected everything. I had always watched others living, but I had limits. Obesity robbed me. It took away my freedom to live life to the fullest. Then, for the first time *ever*, I was ready to put my foot down and change all that. In only twelve months!

I wanted to tackle my weight-loss project the proper way: all natural. This meant no "quick fix" pills, no supplements, no surgery — only by eating the right food combinations (while incorporating all food groups); it was also time to make exercise my new best friend. There's a lot of information out there, but I had to be basically re-educated on food, nutrition, and exercise by my trainer, Robert Lagana. He stripped me of everything I had once thought and believed. This was going to be a brand new beginning for me, what I decided to call my "Complete Body Transformation Project." I knew it would be a difficult challenge, but I was ready.

I decided to go public with my story, hitting up various media, and I even started my very own blog. It was important to me that people have the chance to follow along while my project unfolded, so they might better understand the mental and physical ups and downs one must go through while tackling something like this. It was the best way, I thought, to help and inspire others, to encourage them to take steps in making their *own* lives better also. I wanted to restore any hope they, too, might have lost.

Because of the overwhelming interest in my story, we decided to turn it into book form so we could reach more people. I present you with: *breakin' free.*

RM
December 2008

breakin' free

November 2007

Monday, November 12, 2007

Changing My Body from Obese to . . . ?

Hey there. Tonight I finished taking a shower and sat down to start writing. I would like to introduce myself by saying that I am a Canadian woman who came up with the crazy idea of taking on the challenge of changing my body from obese (275 pounds) to . . . ? in a time period of only 12 months!

The Journey Begins

The reason I left the end blank is because this is the *start* of a journey. Not sure where it will end — I know where I want it to end — but in the meantime, there will be much "in-between" that we have to get through first. I want to share all of it with you! I invite everyone to follow me on this journey. I am hoping to inspire many.

I am thirty-three years old, I'm married with three children, and I work part time. I guess I'm average in that respect. Regarding this transformation idea, I was lucky to have a great trainer/friend/professional bodybuilder hop on board beside me to share his expertise during my personal project. I am so excited to get started! Working together, we are going to prove to everyone, that with the right tools, anyone — if they want it badly enough — can do what I am about to do.

It's going to be amazing to be able to see first-hand changes in my body that I haven't seen — *ever* — to push it as far as it will go — or how far I can take it. Because I am 5'4", my goal is to get down to 125 pounds, with a 20% healthy body fat. Think I can do it? WELL LET'S GO!

Tuesday, November 13, 2007

Where Do I Stand Right Now?

Basic Diet*

What I am doing right now is what my trainer is calling a *Baseline Diet*. What is a basic diet? In my trainer's exact words:

> *"When your body is programmed to store fat, which is what yours is programmed to do, you have to limit yourself to certain foods. This is done so you will have a baseline strategy to determine which foods are causing you to store fat. Everyone is different in this respect. The more overweight you are, the more you have to start eating basics. This re-programming is essential in getting your body back to burning fat. The foods I choose for you are to produce only the most efficient energy during its adjustment back to a fat-burning machine. Once your body responds the way it should, the next stage is to adjust the diet. Whether this means exchanging different foods, or adjusting the ratio of carbohydrates (carbs) to proteins to fats, your diet will be adjusted according to the internal feedback your body is going to give you, along with my professional training experience which we'll use to adjust it in the right way."*

*Carbs — at least 130 grams; Fat — less than 65 grams; Fibre — at least 15–20 grams; Potassium — 4.7 grams; Sodium — 1.5 to 2.4 grams.

My First Day?

So how did I do on my first day, you might be wondering? Well, I am going to tell you. Not bad. A little hungry because I am so used to filling my stomach until it feels full and comfortable. With this diet, there is always room left to still be feeling a little hungry, because now I am eating small meals every three hours, instead of huge ones. (Something I guess I need to get accustomed to.) My energy level surprises me because I feel — even though I am eating differently — that I have a lot of energy!

As far as exercise goes, I am not really expected to do much this month in terms of cardiovascular (cardio) training. I was surprised when I heard *that* one — I guess like the Baseline Food Diet, I will be doing certain exercises using what I think is called a medicine ball, and some weights.

Apparently, these activities will get my body ready for the kick-ass routines which I am sure Rob will plan for me later.

But according to my trainer, I will still lose weight doing those exercises. So, I guess we'll see. However, because I wanted to, I started some cardio. I am walking on the treadmill. This is my own decision. I know I don't have to, but it makes me feel better and gets me in the right frame of mind. Not to mention that I felt so weird not doing anything until this Friday when I meet with Rob and he shows me and walks me through my workout routine.

Overall, I feel good!

Wednesday, November 14, 2007

Morning of My Third Day on the Basic Diet

Last two days felt great: full of energy, hope, smiles . . . Then this morning — all of a sudden — it hit me. A friend has sent me an e-vite for a Christmas party. One of the things highlighted was the FOOD part. *Damn*. I cannot go. This morning I'm just feeling a little weak. I will not cheat, however. I have these pictures in my head at this moment with all BAD stuff. I have to take my daughter and son to the clinic this morning and it's at a local superstore. I am thinking to myself how nice it would be to go into the good part of the store and purchase some really bad foods.

"*Damn*" (today's new word)

Shitty on me man. Oh well. I'm going to make myself go to the gym later this morning so I won't think about this. I was going to skip it for today. However, with me feeling like this, once I bring the kids home, I am heading out there — before I head off to work. Nothing a walk on the treadmill cannot fix. I *hope*.

Friday, November 16, 2007

It's Friday! I Got through the First Five Days

The last two days have been extremely hard on me. Yesterday was my grandmother's wake. I was never good at going to those things. When it was time to leave, I had a quick thought: *It would be nice to drive by a McDonald's drive-through for a Big Mac.* But I got through it. I had to stare at pizza *twice* yesterday (smelled really good), but I didn't taste any. *Yay!*

It's Getting Easier

It's funny. As time moves on, it is actually (believe it or not) getting easier regarding my food. Don't get me wrong, I still miss the smells, I can still remember what the sauces taste like in those great fatty foods, but . . . the cravings seem to pass a lot faster, and I am starting to understand when it's just a craving, rather than thinking I am hungry, and acting on it. My stomach is starting to get used to the food quantities because — I noticed all of a sudden when I stopped to think about it — *I am* NOT *hungry.* Wow! Could this be real? I am so used to feeling hungry that this is something I've never experienced.

Also, surprisingly, I had three people tell me yesterday that I look different. Two said I look like I lost weight, the other said I just look different, I look good. My face, my skin . . . I don't know why that is. Could it be that the natural foods I have been eating are starting to work on my face, my skin? Could it be the thirty minutes of walking on the treadmill? Could it be the excitement of this whole changing idea? Kind of interesting, huh? Makes me wonder . . .

Funny quick story. I went to get my first pictures developed. My gawd! I was . . . I don't even know if embarrassed cuts it — I was pretty shocked to say the least. I mean, let me tell you, huge legs, my ankles are big, I can even see marks that my socks have left. Every little detail. Put it this way, the ONLY and I mean *ONLY* thing I liked about those pictures was my HAIR. Good thing I like to laugh because I really think I should be crying. It's like a friggin' nightmare come true!

Anyway, I went into a local store and had them printed for my own use and of course I see this guy all the time. I go in there to buy the kids' milk and diapers, so all the employees know me well. So I was really nervous, like thinking this guy is going to see my huge legs, my big arms. I mean in the pictures, I am in really short shorts (the shortest I could find) and a tank top, so all my flaws could be seen). But then I just thought *Screw it. I really don't care. Face it. Move on.*

So I walked in with a friend and ordered them.

The man said "Oh. They'll be ready in 20 minutes."

"Sure." Big smiley me thinking *Oh gawd, this man doesn't know what's about to hit him.*

So when we returned, I told my friend "Watch what I'm going to say." (When I'm embarrassed my humour comes out.) So I walk up and say "hey" in a cheery voice (not to mention talking as if I was the sexiest woman alive and so confident. NOT!), smiling: "Are my model pictures ready?" I started laughing my friggin' head off. *Man!* I just didn't want to be there!

I ran out pretty fast. I told him: "You won't have to view pictures like this again for another month. Go have a few drinks and everything will be just fine." I think he thought I was crazy.

That's my funny, embarrassing moment I thought I'd share with you all. And to mention my first pictures are coming up. Thought I'd give you a warning to prepare you. Take a deep breath and I suggest you have a few drinks. Whatever you need to take to relax . Don't be scared and just remember: I am doing this for me. For my trainer. And for all those who think they need to change something, no matter what it is, but think they can't. Because if I can go from 275 pounds (what you are about to see in my photos) to 125 pounds with 20% body fat — that is 150 pounds in 12 months (that's just crazy shit) — then believe me, anyone can make a change! I can? You can. You just have to believe. This is so real. Nothing fake about it. We are all going to witness me changing together. Every month, I will post new photos so you all (including myself) can keep track of how I'm doing. It's going to be an amazing journey.

Saturday, November 17, 2007

Before-Shots: Here Are My First Photos, Taken November 11, 2007

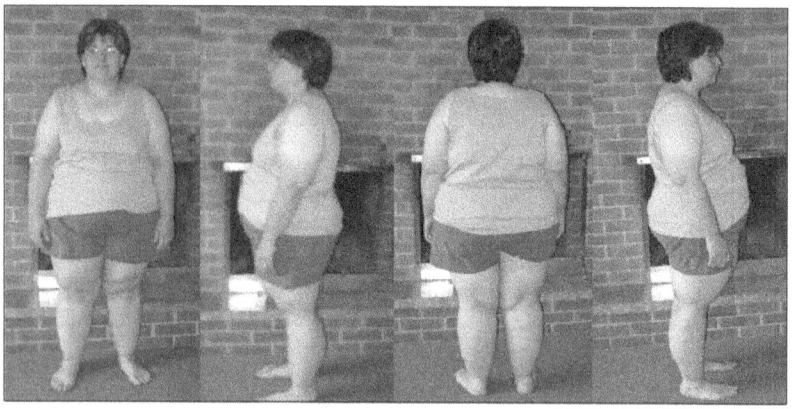

Next photo session: December 11, 2007.

Monday, November 19, 2007

I've Now Finished My First Week (6 Pounds Lighter!)

Finished my first week. Went pretty well.

Last night, however, I came face to face with my worst enemy — McDonald's!

Husband decides to bring home some leftovers from there, that the kids didn't end up eating. WORST MISTAKE EVER! I actually was getting hungry, and there it was . . . sitting there . . . staring at me. So I went up to it . . . I looked at it . . . thought for a split second *What is one bite going to do? Just one bite. My trainer doesn't have to know.* So I picked the hamburger up. I smelled it. I put it down. I picked up a fry. Smelled that. I even rubbed it on my lip while deciding *Am I going to eat this?* At that point, "my drive" that brought me here in the first place, and the thought of how great my body feels eating all the *right* stuff lately, came in to save me from disaster.

I grabbed it and chucked it right into the garbage. I even threw other garbage on top of it. *Phew!* That was close.

And did I ever give my husband a load of shit for doing that. I told him "DON'T EVER BRING THAT JUNK INTO THE HOUSE AGAIN!" (Poor guy.)

But I didn't eat it, thank God. Amazing though, what smells can do.

New Exercise Routine

I met with my trainer on Saturday morning. He showed me my new exercise routine. (See the back of the book for exercise routines.)

A few points I feel I should mention, which helped me get through this week:

1. *Having someone like my trainer behind me as extra pressure.* A trainer who actually takes the time to email me, call me if necessary, and who's basically there any time I need him. One who treats me with respect, believes in me, and provides me with all the RIGHT tools and information.

2. *I am taking it only one day at a time* rather than looking at the long forecast which would discourage me, as it does many.

3. *Gym* — Working out, I think, is so important, not only for the losing weight part, but it makes me feel so relaxed afterwards. Even if I'm stressed going in, I walk out feeling so different. So when it's time to work out, rather than look at it as Oh Gawd, Got To Go To The Gym Again, I try to keep positive. I focus on remembering those feelings I have when leaving, and the feeling of real satisfaction when I am done. I keep my mind on the body I am trying to bring out, the whole purpose of this journey. Something that WILL HAPPEN.

4. *Looking at this as a transformation process* and most of all a learning experience. If I looked at this as just "Another Diet," I think I would have failed already. Instead, this time around, I am looking at it as something interesting, and to take in as much as I can from my trainer. I mean honestly, I am so lucky to have a chance like this. Not to mention for *free?* It's like I am doing a documentary on this topic and using myself as a guinea pig. It's real. Hands on. You see change right before your eyes. Awesome! There is no way to really understand it unless you live it and God knows that is what I am doing, living what

most Canadians and Americans are living every day.

5. *Stop eating the kids' leftovers!* Never mind the money you spent on the food. Never mind that it's good-tasting food. When they are done, throw it out ASAP! This is something I am sure many parents can relate to. Big problem eating whatever the kids leave behind, and doing it for many reasons. Either way, bad habit. Doesn't help in losing weight at all!

Tuesday, November 20, 2007

Today Was a Great Day!

Not sure why, but I had loads of energy which helped a lot at work. One thing I like about my job is that it's physical. (I work as a housekeeper.) Not that it's the best job — although the pay is good — but right now I think this is something that will help me. Any physical extras I can get right now, help.

More on the Ball Lately

I notice myself putting a little more effort into my physical job than before, and I have more on the ball lately because of the energy I have. Instead of looking forward to that time of day — which used to be my favourite (when our cook makes lunch for the employees) — I find myself finding other things to do during what used to be my eating time. Now I just enjoy my own food when I have a moment. My lunch doesn't take twenty minutes like it did before, only a few short minutes because of the smaller quantities I now eat. But I do eat more often. Sometimes it's hard because even *my* food smells good (which makes me want

11

to have more of it). But it's great how I know now that I am actually not hungry. I can finally understand that. Before, my stomach always spoke, and without thinking, I would just eat way too much.

Big Difference in Energy Level
I went to the gym this morning and had a great workout. I went on the elliptical, and I tell you, as time passes I am really noticing a big difference in my energy level, even concerning my daily workouts. It's awesome! At work or home I just find I can do a lot more, I have a certain jump when I am doing my job now, I seem to find myself dancing around sometimes. I think I am smiling more, just happy and easygoing, where before I really didn't have that. Also, when something is thrown my way, I can keep up a lot better than before all this — to think it's only been a little over a week! Wow! Incredible! And I don't even know what I'll feel like later on when I get better and more fit. But right now, I am enjoying every minute with my body as I witness it changing one step at a time.

I spoke to Rob tonight, and we went through my workout for tomorrow, basically recapped it all from last Saturday. I wanted to make sure I had everything down pat before I started, because tomorrow I am tackling my weight training on my own. (In the real world, people have to work. They have families. Obviously, I cannot expect Rob to be by my side every single day, which is good because I want him to see that I can be really strong and dedicated, and can do it alone without my hand being held.) I wrote everything down, and I'm really confident that tomorrow I am going to have an awesome workout!

When Rob took time out to come to the gym for me last Saturday, it was so nice because he walked me through every exercise to make sure I understood everything — from the importance of my posture, to listening to my body, making sure it wasn't too much or wasn't too little. He watched, making sure I was doing the exercises right (he even joined in and did some with me).

I still felt sore two days later, but it was so fantastic. It felt good to feel sore — if that makes any sense — to feel those muscles that I haven't felt in so long, to realize they are still there and haven't vanished! Tomorrow, I'm going to give it my best shot and will continue doing so until I need to change my exercise routine (in five weeks or so). For now, I do three days of cardio, two days of weight training which will be bumped up as we go along, I suppose. And I cannot wait!

Overall, great day! Love my trainer! Everything is working out well.

Saturday, November 24, 2007

Last Weekend before Weigh-In

I must admit that my trainer tells me to stay away from the scales till a month has passed, but I have this obsession (not to mention I'm stubborn as hell), so I like to weigh myself once a week.

By Monday, I will have tackled two weeks.

Friday Night at the Gym Means Young Guys!
Last night after work, I did my weight training at the gym again. I have to say I was a little

uncomfortable at first because I didn't realize that on Friday nights there would be a lot of young guys there. Nonetheless, I got up the courage and went ahead with what I was assigned to do. I still have to learn to let go of wondering what people are thinking when they look at a fat person working out. Who gives a shit! Be strong. Let it go. I will take charge of my own life. If people are going to criticize, so be it.

Last night, I didn't notice anyone who really cared, so that was good. I guess it's more of a mental thing, if anything. One thing I do know, I am not going to let any silly comments — if I get any — hurt my performance. It's not worth it. I pretend I am a model with an excellent body.

Looking "Bad Food" in the Face
I am getting a lot better at looking "bad food" in the face and being near people eating it. Doesn't bother me as much as it first did. I still wish . . . But then I think: *One day I will be able to enjoy the occasional pig-out, it's not the end of the world — and food isn't going anywhere!*

Under the Weather
I'm under the weather at the moment. It started last night. Tonight I have a bit of a sore throat, temperature is up, but it's nothing a couple of Tylenol can't fix.

Also, tonight, I visited my mom and sister who brought up that I look different. Funny, all these You-Look-Different comments from people. They haven't seen anything yet! Must be the four litres of water I'm drinking every day!

Since this transformation process began, I have even let go of *Pepsi!* (*gawd*, I was addicted to that

SO bad), and sugar, and salt. Everything has been damn natural. It's hard to believe how much "bad stuff" we allow ourselves to consume without really knowing what's in it! I know for SURE my skin and body are going to start looking different now that they're not getting any of this unhealthy man-made stuff.

Monday, November 26, 2007

Last Night Was Awful!

And when I say awful, I mean AWFUL. Not sure why, but my nerves were shot. I was really edgy. Maybe it's the weekend thing again because I always find them difficult. Didn't have a chance to work out. Was looking at flyers wondering what I would be making this year for Christmas since I always have it here at my place, with the family. Guess the food just looked way too good. I don't know.

I got through it. Drank lots of water. Cursed a lot. Yelled a lot. Today seems to be getting off to a better start.

Early Gym

I hit the gym this morning at 6:30. I can't believe I got up so early to go to the gym! I don't think I've done that in my entire life!

I figured I'd be better off because on the days I have to do my weight training (now bumped up to three days a week), I find the workout longer. Because I start work at 11:30 a.m., it's better to go in the morning. Weekends aren't good because husband works, etc., so it's more convenient if I go Monday to Friday mornings.

Thank goodness it's only three days a week that I have to be up so early. The other two days, I'll be doing only cardio, so I can be there after 8:00 a.m. because cardio takes only thirty minutes.

It's nice going in the morning. Getting out of my car I was thinking: *Wow. The world is so quiet at this time.*

I also thought there couldn't possibly be many people there, but when I walked in, I was surprised that almost all the cardio treadmills and ellipticals were taken. Pretty good for 6:30 in the morning.

Thankfully, no one is as crazy as I am to do weights at that time of the morning. Half asleep. No breakfast. That's good ol' me.

Getting Better
It was fantastic. The exercises are getting a lot better. I'm getting to know them fairly well, so my form is getting better, I think.

With all this stuff I've been doing, I'm proud to say that I am now 259 pounds. I have lost 16 pounds in my first two weeks!

Yay!

Impossible? No!
Know what's even better? Better than losing 16 pounds? Something that has put a real smile on my face? I can see that already my legs are taking form. That's right! I know you're probably thinking: *"Impossible!"* But it's true! I really think my legs are looking leaner. Not sure if it's the squats or what, but I noticed it this morning. I'm

SO happy. My legs are the worst part of my body, where most of my weight gets stored.

That makes me so happy.

I think I've lost inches in other places, too.

I can't wait till my butt starts looking smaller. Maybe it already has. Not sure. All I know is the leg thing makes me oh so happy.

This working out and watching what I eat is really paying off!

Two more weeks until my next pictures. I have never in my life been so excited to have my picture taken. Usually, I can't stand seeing myself in photos. Now, I can't wait to see what differences a month's worth of working out and healthy eating will show.

Need to go feed the kids. Who knows what they're into while I'm writing.

Wednesday, November 28, 2007

Last Few Days Were Tough

Am fighting off a really bad cold. Damn, I hate colds. However, I'm still going to the gym as usual. Surprised? I don't even know how I've done it, probably because I'm scared *not* to go, that I might start the bad habit of not going. I'm on a roll, I *have* to get there.

This morning was tough because it was another early one. Instead of getting up at 6:00 and getting out the door, it was more like 6:30. For me this is bad, every minute counts in the morning, so-much-to-do-so-little-time type thing. I mean, I have to get my workout in, go back home, get my daughter to school (Senior Kindergarten); then there are the other two children I have to feed, dress, etc; then take my shower, get my meals ready to take with me, make the beds, and there's my writing, too.

Man! Time flies. I never have enough of it.

Killer Weekends

Maybe it's better this way. Right now, my problem is weekends and too much time at home. It's a killer to go through. I find that especially on weekends I get so . . . like . . . I want to eat more, but I can't. Then my nerves start. At least with work, and having a busier week, it takes my mind off things for a while. The days pass more quickly, and before I know it, another five days have gone by.

Staying Away from the Scale

Other than that, things are going well. I'm staying away from the scale until Monday because it doesn't do any good to weigh myself every day. (My trainer is concerned. He says to leave a month between weighings. Yeah, right! Too hard for *moi* to do. If I don't lose that pound . . . I get ANGRY. I think of the hard work I did the day before without losing anything. Funny, eh? Crazy. Monday I'll know where I'm at.

Know What's Interesting?

Next time someone tells you they've lost 10 pounds, think about this. I know it doesn't sound like much, but last night while walking around the fruit and vegetable store, I looked at a bag of potatoes that were 10 pounds. I picked up that bag for fun. Know what? That thing is heavy! So whether it's water I lost, or whatever — for the scale to read 10 pounds fewer . . . Hey. That's a lot of weight, a lot less on a body than it used to carry. Always keep that in mind. It's good to look at it that way.

We don't realize how much we are actually carrying because our bodies get used to the extra weight. It feels normal, we don't know any different, but imagine carrying that 10 pounds, then times that by let's say roughly 15? Wow. That's *heavy*, man! I don't even know how I haven't had a heart attack. (Thank God!)

I will be back on Monday to let you know where I am weight-wise, and then I believe it's one week after that when I'll be posting my One-Month-After-Start pictures. So excited! I mean, I cannot wait to compare! Soon after that, we'll be comparing all those "great measurements" we took in the beginning. We'll learn, in inches, how much I have lost from different areas of my body.

God forbid those measurements have stayed the same after all this hard work I've been putting into this whole transition thing. I think I would just freak out. It would be my worst nightmare come true!

Speaking of nightmares, one quick note: I keep having one that I am always eating Bad Stuff, and saying "Oh, my trainer won't know." There I am stuffing my face. I wonder why I am dreaming that? Perhaps just the thought of failing is always in the back of my head. I don't know.

Friday, November 30, 2007

Friday Night at the Gym . . . Turned Bad!

It's 8:46 p.m. A little late, but I went to the gym after work. I am still sick, can't seem to kick this cold. I have a bad cough and I'm congested, and my throat was hurting today and tonight . . . until I went to the gym. It seems that when I go and work out my throat doesn't hurt anymore. Strange. Maybe it's the heat going on inside that soothes the throat? I'm sure tomorrow morning it'll hurt once again. I think if it does, I'll be visiting a local clinic.

I haven't told you this in depth, but now I HATE going to the gym on Friday nights. But if for some reason I miss in the morning, I have to go at night. Since I woke up today in really rough shape due to my cold, I had to go tonight instead. The Friday-Night-Younger-Guys Crowd act like they're "all that," and make regular people like me feel uncomfortable. They are distracting, they swear, they talk silly.

The workout started off okay. I'm kind of getting used to not caring about what others think — I really am starting to get stronger — so I went ahead and did my warm up, my stretches, and got started on my weight training. But right at the end where I had to do my sets of squats, the last exercise (the hardest to do (not sure if my trainer did that on purpose)), some guy comes over and asks me if I'm finished with the last machine.

I said, "Yeah. Sure. Sorry. Go ahead."

(I'm always apologizing for things. I am also

always polite and I smile when I talk. It's just the way I was brought up.)

He reacted snobbishly. Didn't even comment, but went on to do his own thing.

I thought, *Whatever.* Not sure why he wasn't friendly, but I had other, more important things to concentrate on.

Then his friend comes along and starts talking stupid. At first, I thought he was merely making friendly conversation. He started telling me how his friend is looking good, and how he used to be a lot bigger, that he still has a stomach, but doesn't he look good.

"I guess. Yeah." (Because I wasn't sure where he was coming from.)

He kept jabbering and telling me how he knows his father and that the two are like brothers and that his dad's name is Ben, or something. Then he started laughing. He had a smirk on his face.

So what started off as what I thought was conversation, turned out to be this guy talking stupid with me, laughing.

Well! Didn't *that* turn me the wrong way!

Even though he didn't say anything to hurt my feelings directly, there was something in the way he was talking, the look he was giving his friend . . . The whole situation made me uncomfortable — *angry!* Now that I'm older, I can smell jerks from far away, and I just knew in my mind at that point, okay . . . *Stay away!*

So, the last squats I had to do? Boy, did I do them! I was so angry that he did this to me that I ended up taking it out on my legs (a good thing now that I look back) but it left me feeling sad.

When I was doing my cool-down on the treadmill later, I thought: *Why isn't my trainer here with me? If he was here, they wouldn't have talked to me like that. Why were they laughing? Were they laughing at me? Was that guy just being sarcastic with me for fun? To have a laugh? At least what he thought was fun?*

At one point, I put my head down while walking on that treadmill because I thought I was going to cry. Strange how that got to me. I started off on a high, then all of a sudden, I hit an all-time low!

Not Even Hedley Could Help

Once I got into my car, not even my favourite group Hedley that I always listen to on my CD player, could get me out of that quiet stage. I found myself rehashing the whole scenario. I was quiet, feeling sad, upset. That's one thing I am going to have to learn not to do. I tend to think a lot, and sometimes over-analyze things. I should not have let a petty thing like that get to me.

But driving home, I couldn't help thinking about that whole situation, and it started bringing back memories and things I have been through in the past. I wasn't going to write about them but hey, might as well write a couple, at least.

Grade 7: A time when kids are plain old mean. This one guy and his friend, every time I took a step, would make these noises. *Boom boom boom boom.* It was something I'd seen in movies, but this was happening to *me*. They would call me Chunky.

I can still hear those two boys in my mind: "Chun-ky. Chun-ky. Chun-ky."

Gawd. Makes me tear up just thinking about it. I held that memory inside for so long. I never even thought about it again until tonight. I never told anyone about it or how it made me feel. The only people who knew were the people in my class who would hear it as well. None of them would stick up for me. I guess everyone had their own issues to worry about.

I also remember another time. I went to a party with a girlfriend (at the time) and her boyfriend. When I got there with them, the friend having the party (the host), looked at them and at me at the door and said in Italian (not realizing I'm Italian) "Why did you bring this cow?"

Yup. That's what he said.

I remember feeling shocked. At the time I wasn't even big like now.

(I have to pause here, sit back for a moment, not believing I have opened up about these memories, that they are now written on the screen before me.)

I suppose there are a lot of stored memories inside me. People know me as a friendly person, always smiling. In high school, I always had really cute guys as friends, but yet . . . like many, I had my share of sadness throughout my years.

If anything tonight, those guys just brought it all back. I left the gym feeling so sad. Unless people have been in my shoes and have been overweight, they can never understand how those remarks just kill.

Being overweight is so terrible, because it's not something you can hide. It's reality. It's right out there for all to see.

Determined!

Anyway, I don't want to talk any more about this depressing stuff. I will leave it at that for tonight. All I know is that I am feeling stronger. I am determined not to fail. I made it to the gym tonight, without supper, in blizzard-like weather, lots of snow, and sick. So if that doesn't tell you how determined I am, I'm not sure what would.

My trainer and I are going to be on a local programming channel soon, and I have a lot of stuff to look forward to.

My Trainer — An Angel

I love my trainer. I cannot speak more highly about anyone. He has helped me believe I can do this, that it's not that bad. He is so fantastic to talk to. I know he's going to be there every step of the way because that's the kind of person he is, he would never leave me hanging. He is positive and a believer, sweet, understanding. He is there for me, and I feel it. I guess we were meant to meet up again.

He was someone I went to school with but never actually got close to. I think this is a project that, if nothing else, will bond us. I think I'm going to learn much from him and from this experience. I also believe he will learn something from this and from me as well.

I want to prove to him that I can do it, that I can follow direction, and most of all I want him to see me, and see all the changes he will help me make, because in the end, it takes both me and him working together. I need his experience, his own years of hard work, and he needs me to actually physically change by following his directions, because the end result will be what we both put into this. He hasn't worked with anyone in the weight category I'm in, so I am sure this is a great project for him as well, and you'd better believe I'll be letting people know about him! He's a person who deserves every bit of success from this, from every standpoint.

I will never forget what he told me: Even if I just needed his help to change, with no publicity involved, he would still have done it for me for free anyway, because it's his passion. And you know what? I really believe that! It shows what kind of man he is. (My angel.)

Getting way too sensitive about things tonight, aren't I? Tomorrow is a whole new day. Looking forward to the scale on Monday.

December 2007

Sunday, December 2, 2007

December Already!

Can't believe we're already in December! (Although the snow we've been having reassures us that yes, we *are* in December.)

I Can Deal with Weekends Now!

I would like to mention one good thing. This past weekend has been great in one way. I can deal with the weekends now I guess. I didn't feel hungry this weekend, or on edge like all the other weekends that have passed. It didn't bother me and I wasn't really hungry much anyway. Yesterday, I had to force myself to actually *eat* the foods I'm supposed to take in every day. So that is a GOOD thing. I hope all weekends will now be this way! I can enjoy my kids more and not be so miserable.

Tomorrow I'll reveal my weight!

Monday, December 3, 2007

Drum Roll Please!

I'M 16 POUNDS LIGHTER! *Yay!*

In three weeks, I have lost 16 pounds!

How do I feel? (Other than being still sick?) I feel more energetic, I can run up the stairs at home without being all out of breath like in the beginning, I smile a lot more, and I am starting to feel stronger both mentally and physically. I have overcome temptations and I don't have a problem being around them anymore. I feel more in control over what's going into my mouth instead of always out of control (letting food control ME).

I feel wonderful. I am excited about next week's pictures. I hope they show some change. I know the changes won't be huge, but I do expect a little. I'm going to work out hard this week, and next week, after the 11th, you can see my pictures. Together, we can try to find the differences like we used to in kindergarten.

Remember! These pictures are temporary, they are going to change all the time. Life goes by so fast, before you know it, I'll be posting my three-month pictures.

Tuesday, December 4, 2007

We're Going to Be on TV!

I am really excited to announce that my trainer and I are going to be on a local station here in Ottawa once a month until the end of this journey. It's on Rogers local channel 22, the program is called "Daytime." I hope that whoever can, will check us out.

This morning I went to the gym. I had to do my training despite the fact I am still coughing but I had no choice. At first I had a rough time with coughing fits, and needing water because of that. Wasn't sure if I was going to get through it, but the coughing passed and I was able to get through today's training. Can't wait until this cough goes away. (With the kids, I expect another one sooner or later. Hopefully, later.)

Thursday, December 6, 2007

"Dealing"

I've had a really tough day today. Not sure why, but I was very hungry. I was at work, and time seemed to go by so slowly I could hardly wait for my time to eat lunch, and snacks. That's all I could think about!

I really don't know why that happened. Perhaps I put more into my workout this morning? My trainer had given me the heads up that I might feel hungry, and that it would be normal. He told me to stay strong, we'll be changing my diet soon, but I have to be strict right now on my basic diet to get things started off right. But that was three weeks ago! I thought I wasn't going to have to deal with that. Well . . . Today I dealt with it!

I hope I will be over it by tomorrow, because it was tough at work, smelling the foods around me.

I told Mike, the chef, at work how I was feeling, while chowing down on my grapes (when the others were eating potatoes, meat, and veggies), so he said: "Drink your water. You haven't been drinking your water. Drink your friggin' water!"

I like him. He's the type to tell it like it is. He's not too soft with me which I think is what I need right now. I'd rather someone be hard on me, and not feel sorry for me (or give me the impression that they're feeling sorry for me). I really think he doesn't want to see me do anything I will regret. I have come so far in just a month.

He said: "Your trainer's not here, but I am, and I'm telling you to drink!" It worked! I drank down a few glasses and it helped a lot. (But I have to say diets really suck! I know I really shouldn't call it a "diet," but anything that leaves me feeling hungry I call a diet.)

The cook and I have had a lot of conversations about this. He's been the one to listen to me, not only on this topic, but on a lot of topics. He's become a friend and confidant. He was there when I received the call from Rogers television, he knows how excited I was, and how excited I have been. He's helped me stay strong as well. Thanks to him, I got through the day a little easier. In the end, it's all up to me — or you, or whoever the person is, going through whatever situation. I mean friends can help support you, but you in the end make that final decision on what's going to go into that mouth.

Holiday Season . . .

I think this coming holiday season is going to be hard on me. Although my trainer told me I can eat whatever on Christmas Day, honestly I am scared to do so. It's been almost a month that I have not had things like sugar, salt, pasta, et cetera, and I have been eating so healthily that if I have a taste of *one* of those things . . . What if it starts me craving things? What if it triggers something in my brain that puts me in an even worse position? I don't want to go through that again!

There will be plenty of time to enjoy those things from time to time later on down the road. Do I really want to take a chance with this and risk all I've done so far? Right now I might be hungry, but it's not like I am *craving* things. There's a difference.

I'm beginning to think about what I am going to do over the holidays. Maybe I'll avoid the whole

31

thing altogether and just treat it like a normal day. That would be hard to do as well, because when you have a family (including three kids under the age of five), how can you possibly treat Christmas like just another normal day.

Christmas is in the air, baked goods, lots of Italian food, turkey, potatoes, gravy, the whole nine yards. Okay. I'd better stop. I'm making myself hungry here. Again.

Good Thoughts

Today I was thinking some good thoughts, as well, while I took in some air outside at work, while trying to deal with my hunger.

I did have a minute to think about what I HAVE accomplished in the past month of training and transformation. I have made it to the gym four weeks in a row, at least five times a week. I have not cheated once. I have followed all the instructions given to me by my trainer. I can now climb the stairs in my own house without being out of breath. I have much more energy at work. I have increased some of my weights because some of the exercises are getting easier (I'm challenging myself on my own while my trainer's away). There's a big difference compared to when I started.

I think I should always focus on and remember these things. A year from now isn't that far away. Not really. Time flies so fast . . . Before I know it, I'll be at the finish line, weighing over 100 pounds less. I wonder how I'll feel when I get there. I mean I have never *ever* been a normal weight. Not since maybe Grade 2?

I don't even know what it feels like to be a normal weight. I was always overweight! Isn't that sad. All these years I missed out on so much because of it. I guess the good thing is, I'm tackling it now. Better now than never, and I still have a lot of years left to enjoy my new me once I get there. I can't wait to get it all off once and for all.

Friday, December 7, 2007

Some Barrels to Leap

I have a few barrels to get over these next few weeks.

Tomorrow is my daughter's fifth birthday. Everyone (big family) is coming for a nice fresh, sweet-icing princess cake I'll probably want to devour, and chips and nachos with a dip I'm making with sour cream and fresh chopped tomatoes, green onions, shredded cheese, and black olives; thick crust pizza smelling oh-so-good with all the dressings, and melted cheese on top, and nice ice-cold pop. God help me.

. . . then the following week I have to go through the same ordeal when it's my nephew's birthday at my brother's house. God help me twice!

. . . then there will be Christmas. (I am beginning to think this was a really shitty time to start a transformation diet.)

Monday, December 10, 2007

Good for Me!

. . . the birthday party for my daughter? I passed the test with flying colours! I had not one bite of *any*thing, not the delicious mouth-watering pizza, not the sweet cake that I ordered (the one everyone kept mentioning was so good), not even the amazing nacho dip with the crunchy nachos that I made for everyone. I am SO pleased with myself about this. I stuck to my own food. To be honest, the whole thing didn't bother me as much as I thought it would!

GOOD FOR ME!

As far as my weight goes, I guess I'm having what would be a "Biggest Loser" moment: The numbers on my scale did not move this week AT ALL! I was really hoping to get to 20 pounds today since it will be exactly a month tomorrow; and it would have been nice to have an even number. But no. Nothing. *Nada. Niente.*

Am I upset? A little. But I have better things to be happy about. I have done all that I could do. I have not cheated. Best of all, my trainer will be back at the end of this week. We'll meet and have an "oil change" done on my routine —change of menu, change of exercises — to keep my body shocked and on target. I'm looking forward to that! I have been on this basic diet now since I started November 11. (Yes, I'm used to it, but I think it's time for a change!)

The exercises at the gym have, like I said, been getting easier. (Mind you, some are still difficult, and I'll never get used to, or like, those, e.g., squats, but I'm ready to start a new bunch of exercises!)

The city editor from the *Ottawa Sun* got in touch with me over the weekend, and it's set! During the week of December 31, they have decided to run an ad, have a first picture, talk about what I'm trying to accomplish, and then follow my story for a year! Amazing. They will be posting video clips of me training, and of me talking on their website where people can go to see me and what I'm up to (pictures updated every month!). I can't wait to tell my trainer all about this!

I wanted to inspire, and it looks like it's going to happen now that everyone will have access to my story, and see who I am.

Tomorrow, my "famous" pictures!

Tuesday, December 11, 2007

One Month Anniversary!

I have to say that I, personally, am very pleased with my pictures. I got emotional this morning posting them because it all hit me. All those mornings I was getting up early, working out hard, resisting temptations throughout this past month — just everything! and when I saw my photos I was really surprised! Honest. I didn't think they would show that much of a difference yet. *Wow.*

Can't wait to see what surprises lie ahead for *next* month. And every month thereafter, because I'm going to keep posting them until I'm done.

It's been really hard, I cannot lie, but, in the end it's so worth it! It's a feeling I just can't explain in words other than to say I feel like I'm on top of the world, like I've overcome something difficult, and am now enjoying the fruits of it all. (And more killer workouts!)

But I would not have changed one thing this past month, and I hope this shows everyone that with the right workouts and proper food intake, anyone can change!

November   *December*

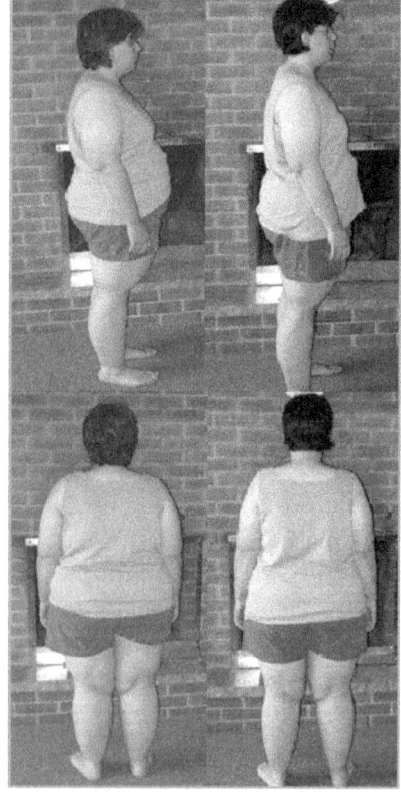

See what only 20 pounds can do? Doesn't sound like much, but look! I hope my trainer is going to be proud. He hasn't seen me since he showed me my routine at the gym. (He returns this Sunday.) I am so grateful. Rob, it worked! You are my saviour, my friend! Thank you! Now let's kick this thing into high gear. I'm done with the beginner part . . .

Check this out. My neckline in the back, my arms from behind, my butt is smaller, and my hips (and I think I feel tears coming on). I am so shocked that I have changed already this month. (Okay, now I *am* crying, but in a good way.)

November   December

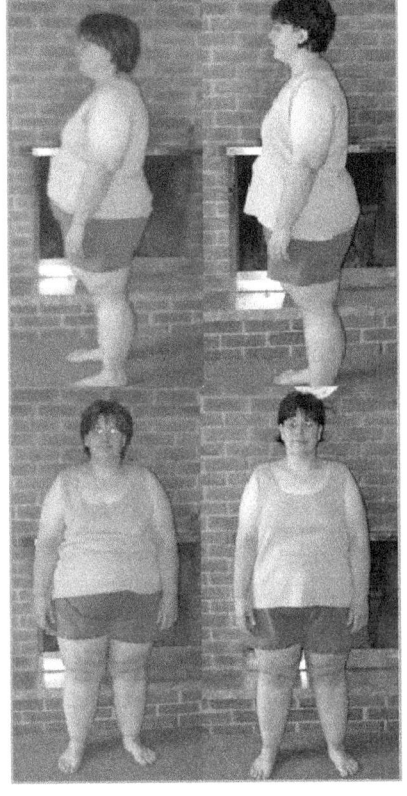

Look at my side view. My stomach doesn't look as big, my arms have gotten smaller, my chin . . . It's all good! I'm feeling really proud at this moment.

So these are my pictures. What a difference! I can't believe it. Never mind that I lost 20 pounds on the scale . . . Pictures really do say it all. All my hard work has paid off. I just need to keep it up. I am *pumped.*

Friday, December 14, 2007

My Body Is Much Stronger

Another week of working out is over. I'm happy with that. I always look forward to my weekends where I don't have to wake up at 5:45 a.m. to get to the gym for 6:00.

It was nice this morning though, because again I can see and feel my body is much stronger than when I started. As I was finishing my exercises, one by one, while putting the weight pieces back in their proper places, I thought to myself, *Wow. I've done it!*

Who knows what the next stage will be like. Not sure if I'll be using these same weights. I might be doing a whole new range of exercises! It was a great feeling though. I can't wait to see my trainer, Rob, so *he* can see how far I've come.

Since I started, there's this one exercise called a bridge, where I have to lie on the ground and lift my whole body up, and hold, and down, and up, and down, et cetera. I had to do fifteen repetitions, three sets, and believe me, that was *tough!* But today, even *that* exercise I went though like a breeze — well not "breeze," but it was easier to do than when I started out. I still have a hard time with squats. They're difficult! But everything else was perfect. My arms are much stronger, my posture is better — even when just standing. (You can see from my photos I am standing straighter.)

After taking pictures of myself on Monday, I almost feel like not weighing myself anymore, Pictures say it all. I look forward to my next set, on January 11.

Monday, December 17, 2007

Weigh-In Day

I didn't want to weigh myself today because the last pictures had such an impact on me. But I figured I would for you guys since I've been doing this every Monday since the beginning.

Today the scales showed about 247, roughly 23 pounds now. From 270 that's pretty good.

38

You know when the dial comes around and shows your weight? Soon, I won't see the "270." It will be out of sight.

Wednesday, December 19, 2007

TV Show Debut

Yesterday was our debut on the television show. It was exciting, however I have to say I was nervous. Before going on I must have gone to the bathroom mirror a million times, checking to make sure I had nothing on my teeth, making sure my lipstick was just right. Usually, I'm not one to fuss about those things, but in a case like this . . .?

All in all, it went okay. The day itself was rushed, and it was an emotional roller coaster. After finishing up at Rogers TV, I had to run over to my uncle's wake. Exactly! I went from the top of the world with excitement, to a really depressing state. It was hard. I had not eaten all day. But I got through it!

Brrr

It's been pretty cold here, which is making it tough for me to get to the gym at 6:00 a.m. I *do* get there, but it takes me about fifteen minutes to convince myself to get out of bed. I lie there, and debate, and think *I'm so tired. Do I have to? Could I stay five more minutes? Brrr, it's cold out.* (Every excuse I can think of to stay nice and cozy.) Then finally, I just get up. Grumpy. But I get up. That's the hardest part of this whole thing right now, getting up so early, especially after my kids go to bed so late sometimes. I'm not always operating on a lot of sleep.

For example, this morning when I was doing my weight training — when it should have been waking me up — I found myself yawning a lot. Total opposite!

Something else funny (not sure if anyone can relate): When I'm on the treadmill on my weight training days, I must look like I'm half drunk because I still cannot get used to it. When I walk, I tend to slowly veer to one side, then I have to straighten myself up in the centre again. I just laugh. (I never liked the treadmill, but on the days I'm using weights, I use it to warm up.)

We'll be making monthly appearances on the show and presently, I'm in the process of getting things done before we have the first article in the *Ottawa Sun*, January 2. I have the reporter scheduled to come tomorrow to meet with me, and to take pictures maybe. I'm really excited about that! This has turned into something much bigger than what I'd anticipated. They are even going to show me training on their website, and probably talking into the web cam, et cetera. So even if you are not from where I live, everyone will be able to check it out, and can see me working my butt off. I will keep you posted.

I Love the Challenge

But it's not easy, I tell you, making time for all this. It's hard enough making time to work out, to have time for family, and work, appointments, kids' swimming. Now I have to add this in. It's something I'm still trying to get used to. But I love it. I love the challenge. I love that all of a sudden my once-so-ordinary life is different! And I think we all need that sometimes. Change, I think, can make us stronger, and it gets our brains going again.

I am determined to do this so you can follow my story as I hope to show that people — even people like me who started off so heavy — can change, even if you are a mom, and married, and work. It's not easy, but it can be done. We have the power in our hands to change whatever we wish, pretty much. It's just a matter of grabbing onto it, and getting through it even if it's tough, because in the end, it's SO worth it. I had a taste of it looking at my one-month photos. I can't even imagine what I will be feeling in the end

The main thing I hope to achieve, when I've reached my goal, when I'm physically healthy (a completely different person than the one who's writing right now), is that whoever follows my journey by reading my words — even if you don't have a weight problem — will know that we as people can defeat whatever might need to be defeated! If I can lose 150 pounds . . . Well, I mean . . . It just shows you, as long as you stay strong and positive, and have support from friends and family, and have the right tools, you can reach for any dream and attain it, whatever it is.

It's all about "control." We need to take control of our own lives. That's the key. God made us a lot stronger than we realize, and we should always (me, too) remember that.

The one thing that these sad deaths also have reminded me of is, we have only one life. We choose what we want to make of it.

Freedom!
I have chosen the path to freedom! To live my life without the worries I once had. It feels GREAT! I mean, really, all these years of wasted time? I should have done this a long time ago.

41

I can't believe all these years I just let it go. And go. And go. And for what? Because I like food too much? I mean, come on! I just needed — I think — someone to show me the RIGHT path. Thanks to my trainer, I have found that path.

I will never go back to how I was, how I thought: *Well, this is not a big deal. So what! I'm overweight. Whatever.* But you know what? I was fooling myself. Being overweight made me lose out on a lot. Sadly, some of those things I cannot get back. But I can change the future.

Stay warm. Monday will be another weigh-in day, and before you know it, I will be taking my third set of pictures. *Wow.*

Sunday, December 23, 2007

Decisions, Decisions . . .

Two more nights to decide: Whatever am I going to do about Christmas dinner?

This might be a good time to do some writing because I have something I'm fighting with.

I was safe from having Christmas dinner until Mom called us all and said we are going ahead with the Christmas dinner despite the two deaths that we had to deal with recently.

Starting tonight, I've really been thinking about what I am going to do:

1. Am I going to indulge for the one night?
or
2. Am I going to stay away and just eat my own foods?

42

It's a very difficult decision and let me explain why.

Reasons Why I Should *Eat at Christmas*
- I have been doing so well, that I know, weight-wise, one night would not hurt me.
- I have been strong and have kept up with my challenge to change my body, not cheating once in seven weeks, so I think I deserve to have one night of whatever I want.
- I am going to have to do this sooner or later. I cannot be afraid of the odd day that comes up such as birthdays, anniversaries, New Year's, Christmas. I'm only human. I have to learn control.
- I should just do it, get it out of my system, then get back on track the next day starting with the gym in the morning.

Reason Why I Feel I Shouldn't
- What if that one taste brings back those evil cravings again?
- What if I cannot regain control, and all of a sudden I get weak?
- What if I can't stop? (I have to ask myself: Do I really want to even *try* this?) To perhaps allow my body to start all over again with those terrible cravings for chocolate, pasta, bread, fried stuff, sweet stuff, cakes, MCDONALD'S?

What to do? I don't know what I'm going to do. All I know is, either way, that night is not going to be a good one. I will have to face all of my family eating, while I'll be eating my own stuff. Or, I might eat for that one night, then deal with the feelings of guilt — and who knows *how* my body will physically react to it, perhaps get sick? All for that one night of indulging.

43

Tonight I am thinking about it so much that it's making me want chocolate and all those foods I know will be there. Sometimes life sucks!

Funny thing is, I went to McDonald's the other day with my mom, while Christmas shopping, and I brought my own food there for lunch. At first, I was really proud and I thought, *This is great to have control over myself for once, not let those foods get hold of me and ruin me like they once did.* I mean who do you know who brings her own chicken sandwich to McDonald's?

But then I looked around, and I realized I was starting to get angry watching everyone eat Big Macs, and fries, and all that stuff. I don't know why I was so angry. After being happy, I was getting this face on me of anger. Why do I have this problem? Why can't I be one of those people who can just eat and eat and eat and not gain a pound? Weird. I think all this Christmas stuff is getting to me. All this shopping, and with our family being Italian, Christmas is not the same without the food! Everyone looks forward to the food. Never mind the presents.

I have to remember one thing: Since I've regained control of what goes into my mouth, now I have time to enjoy simple things like watching my own kids eat, without wanting more, or in this case, nothing of theirs. Sounds strange, but it's true. I never did that before because food just takes over one's thoughts. That's all one is thinking about. Eating. *Man!* Looking back, that is scary. Today, now that my head and stomach don't say "FOOD" all the time, it leaves me with more time to enjoy different little things, whereas before, food controlled everything!

This is a choice I'm going to have to make myself. No one will make that one for me. All I know is, no matter what happens, I will not only tell you all about it, I will come out on top! Whatever decision I make regarding that night, I will live with it, and the next day will be a whole new day. Either way!

I AM going to win this battle. I AM going to be a healthy, more confident person after all this. I will be so different that people won't even *recognize* me. I may not even recognize myself!

This is definitely the toughest challenge I have ever had to face in my life. And lately, with all this thinking about the Christmas feast I'm going to have to confront, I find myself looking in the mirror wondering if I DO look smaller, like I once thought I did. With all this thinking going on, with the thoughts of foods that I haven't had in a long time, I feel I look like the same person before losing all that weight. Isn't that strange how your emotional side can totally change how you perceive yourself? As though that woman from before I started is back again. The one who never exercised, the one who ate whatever she wanted, the one who didn't take responsibility, the one who took the easy way out.

All this negative thinking about food is affecting how I see myself. Is that crazy? It's real, yet I believe now (I think I just realized something new!), when you hit a bump in the road, for whatever reason that might be, you find yourself seeing the *old* you, as you were, when you started, before even losing any weight, along with the negative thoughts that went with that view. I believe this is most probably why I and many others failed in the past. You basically give up, almost like it's not worth the hassle, it's easier eating what's fast and simple.

No one ever said life was easy. If you want something badly enough, you have to work hard for it. We need to remember: Even though it might feel like it's far away right now, it's really not, and when it's done, you'll finally be free. I will have fought the demon that got me here!

Tuesday, December 25, 2007

Four More Hours until I'm Face to Face with the Christmas Feast!

I've made up my mind about what I'm going to do regarding dinner tonight with the family. But I'm not going to reveal it yet.

I chose to do what I'm about to do regarding the dinner because I felt that this was the best decision for me; and that it only made perfect sense to me. *Not even* my trainer knows exactly what my decision is. All he knows is that my emotional state hasn't been the greatest. We have exchanged a few emails regarding tonight, and all I know is, the dinner tonight is going to be amazing! He has given me the okay to eat a good meal if I feel like I need to. He said I should remember to just eat for one and not for two, to stay away from junk (meaning chocolate) . . . (That's funny, Rob. As if!)

I have to look forward to facing a family dinner which consists of: cannelloni, meatballs, breaded chicken cutlets, salad; and I believe we are also going to have turkey, gravy, mashed potatoes, veggies, lots of chocolates, vanilla cake (plus desserts like Mom's pies), wine, Coke, assorted nuts, and God only knows what else. I suppose, this is what being Italian is all about. Food *overload!* And with all the great healthy choices to make? . . . NOT!

My mind *is* set. I am ready to go through it. I will let you all know later what I chose to do. I'll also let you know how I feel about the decision I'll have made, and how I'm feeling in general.

I am making a promise to myself that I will not regret what I choose for tonight, and to remember that the next day, the sun will shine once again, and Christmas will have come and gone.

I CAN tell you however, that this has been extremely hard on me. I've probably been thinking about what was I going to do for the last three days, going back and forth with decisions, thinking of the pros and cons. No wonder I've had emotional breakdowns. Not to mention all these Christmas preparations, stress shopping, and foods, and choices. It's all had a big impact on why I've been feeling the way I have.

I can't even explain, but I will say this is the first time I've found Christmas to be so hard, the MOST DIFFICULT time during this transformation journey so far. I've found myself crying more. Even when writing emails to my trainer.

But this is part of life, the life of someone who's going to make a difference, someone who's looking to inspire, who chose to make this journey public so anyone can follow along to know what I'm going through trying to get to the finish line. I cannot be fake. I have to stay real and continue being honest with all of you.

I will finish this for now until I get back home from "The Dinner," when I reveal what I've decided to do. To be concluded later . . .

To My Trainer

I would *never* be where I am right now, if it weren't for YOU. You are MY angel, who has come along to save ME. Already, in just a short time, you've made me see there's a way to change, that there's a light at the end of the tunnel. Most importantly, you have given back to me the "hope" that was once lost.

Although it's been hard (a whole new learning experience), in just seven weeks I've changed, both physically and emotionally. You've been my strength, you've inspired me . . . And you are such a kind-hearted person that I can't help but feel fortunate to have you once again in my life, after losing contact for many years. I'm so lucky to have YOU by my side, one of the best! By teaching me all your secrets, from your own knowledge, you have given me all the tools I need to conquer this demon, once and for all.

This has been a really tough starting journey, but with you next to me (not always physically, but always there in the background, cheering me on, genuinely caring, having faith in me that I can do it (where others may not have)), makes it easier and keeps me smiling.

Thank you for reading my emails, for caring, and responding so quickly when I need you; for all the phone calls, and checkups, and most importantly for just being you. I hope to make us both proud at the finish line, saying WE DID IT, and WE DID IT RIGHT!

We can show an example to so many others who might also have lost hope . . . to allow them to see that anyone can make a change, that it's all about making a choice and sticking to it, even when it seems impossible.

I will *never* forget what you are doing for me, and I will always be forever grateful.

Okay. I'm Home
It's 9:54 p.m., Christmas night. I must say, I'm relieved to be back home tonight to continue this.

It was tough. The food was amazing, smelled great, looked great, and there was lots of it!

I had my mind made up beforehand that I WAS NOT, repeat, WAS NOT going to have *any* of it! So you can all be relieved.

I hope I scared everyone. God knows I scared myself. I was oh-so-close to giving in for Christmas. The perfect excuse to do so.

I did fantastic. I beat the odds. Not even one bite! How do I feel? Wonderful. I have never had this kind of power over myself in a long time (perhaps never, actually). And because I beat this tonight, I'm sure it will help me down the line when facing another battle.

Actually, it didn't bother me at all! I passed on everything, including the sweet stuff. All this anxiety that I had for the last few days, the thoughts of should I or shouldn't I? how will I be able to pass on that stuff? was I ready to pass on it? would I get weak? All that worry was for nothing. I suppose my trainer has trained me well.

It's all a mind thing, I guess. My body is so used to the good stuff now, that *I'm* used to taking it in. I actually enjoy my own food.

I'm not going to lie. Until this morning, I was so going to go nuts on everything tonight. Not sure why? Maybe because it would have made things so much easier to just give in.

But after speaking to one of my sisters (God bless her), and really talking about it this afternoon, I said, "You know what? You're right. Not even worth it!"

She gave me the last bit of courage I needed to look at it from a different point of view.

I have a transformation project that I need to complete! And not even Christmas is going to stop me from getting to my goal. There's always next Christmas when I'm sure I'll be enjoying all the great foods. But right now, I'm just striving to be my best, both physically and emotionally. Going back to negative eating, even on a day like today, would not have helped me at all, so therefore there was no point in going down that path tonight. Why? For one night? Doesn't make any sense when I've been pushing my body for the last seven weeks to be totally opposite. All those mornings in the gym at 6:00 a.m., my cardio being a hundred times better than when I started, the strength in my body compared to when I first began. NO WAY!

Nothing is going to stop me from reaching for what I want. I can smell it coming, and feel it coming in my gut! And you know what? I DESERVE THIS! High fives everyone!

Monday, December 31, 2007

New Year's Eve — A Day at the Gym with Me

(Something you would see on the Comedy network?)

Happy New Year to you all!

All I can say is: What a day! From start to now. What a friggin' day!

This morning started off rough:

Got up. . . . 6:00 a.m. . . . Ready to leave. Had to use my husband's car (mine's in the shop). Got out there. Start it up. Reverse. Stalls. "Damn."

Try again. Start it up. Reverse. Stalls. "Okay. Now I'm getting mad!"

One more time. Start it up. Reverse. STALLS! GAWD DAMN! Now I'm swearing like there's no tomorrow!

Then the door wouldn't shut. *"Fer chrissake!"* Slam it. Slam it. Slam it. . . . Finally door catches and shuts. And then to end it all, I look down at my hand and notice I have all this thick white oil that looks like lard and smells like some disgusting cheap perfume. My husband has decided to put this on the door to keep the latch from freezing (because sometimes he thinks he's a mechanic. Yeah right). *Nice. This is* GREAT!

So I give up. I get out of the car. Go back into the house. SLAM the door. I am NOT HAPPY. Not happy at ALL!

I am just thinking to myself: *Today I am supposed to tackle my new routine. I don't have a car to go to the gym with.* ISN'T THIS MY LUCKY DAY! Too much snow to bike there. Buses, not sure. Haven't taken one in years. So I call my good old dad . . .

So Dad comes, gives me a lift, and there I am, finally, two hours later, still no breakfast, but ready to tackle my new routine. I took a breather. And started.

First of all, the new balance thing I'm doing makes me laugh. (We've changed it a little, I'm higher than usual, so it's quite funny.) People probably were wondering what in the world is this girl up to now, but I continued. It's all good. Trust what my trainer tells me. So I continued on even though I probably looked like I was practising for the part in *Titanic* where they're at the bow of the ship.

Next, I started on my other exercise which was going fantastic until I felt my knee crack. "*Uuuh.* That can't be good," (shaking my head). So I had to wait. Once I continued, and changed my position a bit, it was okay, but meanwhile, I didn't want to look like a fool — I was sure all eyes were on me, so I had no choice but to continue.

Then for my workout . . . My gosh. Talk about a laugh! There I was, going from one exercise to another — and I swear there was music in the background, to *Rocky*, or some crazy-ass movie, and here I was the star of the show!

So here I am jumping from one thing to another. One minute I'm on the floor. Another, I'm doing legs. Another, doing arms. Oh my *gawd*. I was laughing my head off just thinking about what these other people must be thinking. Not to mention that my trainer expects me to do this *four* times!

Then. To top it all off — when I'm doing my push ups — my boob decides to fall out of my sports bra. Thank God I noticed before I turned around to face everyone (because today I decided to wear my white shirt which is a little revealing if this sort of thing happens). I fixed it all back up, and then *that* was worrying me: *Oh my* gawd, *what if it falls out again?* So I'm running around, constantly feeling to make sure everything is staying where it should. Didn't look too good, I guess.

Don't think I'll be buying a sports bra from a big discount chain ever again. (The things we do to save money!)

Anyway, I felt good when it was all over . . . and kind of happy. It was quite the rush from the previous program, and I really think I am going to love it later.

One more thing: When I was cooling off on the bike (of course, smiling, thinking of what I'd just been through) this little chubby guy who was on a weight machine for legs (God bless him), decided to sneeze so huge — all over his hand — then to give it just a quick wipe onto his clothes and continue on, touching the machine. Made me think . . . *hmm* . . . I see now why I am always getting sick lately . . .

That was my episode at the gym today.

And . . . I am proud to say, I have reached 30 pounds in my weight loss now.

January 2008

Tuesday, January 1, 2008

Happy New Year!

Another year has come and gone. The years go by fast, don't they? The question is, what are YOU going to be doing differently this year? Everything we do in life counts for something. If we all looked back at the path we have started, would we all be proud of ourselves? Would we be able to say that we have done everything that we wanted to do, and in the right way, and in the way we wanted? We're all here for such a short time (only God knows how long, it could be years, days, or even minutes), it's up to us what we do with that time.

Many New Year's Days have come and gone in my life. In the past, I would start a New Year's resolution only to weaken. But this one is going to be different! I am NOT going to let the rest of my years (or days, or minutes) be controlled by food as I did in the past. I've made a firm decision. I'm making a promise to myself this year, to open myself up, to become a stronger individual, both emotionally and physically. To try new things that I was once afraid of trying. To enjoy life, and my friends, and my family, and those I feel close to, and to appreciate the time I have with them.

I want to *surpass* any expectations I might have right now of what "I believe" I can do, and go beyond the Trying My Best Possible mode. I want to challenge my body and mind on a whole new level, push my body the furthest I can possibly push it!

Life can get boring at times, so it's nice to challenge ourselves. It feels great! (Take it from someone who *never* challenged herself before.) We are a lot stronger than we give ourselves credit for. The choice is always ours. It's put into our hands to decide what route we'll take next. *We* have the ability to change whatever we want, whatever's important to us.

Before I started this project, you would never have caught me saying these words to anyone. You would have caught me eating the way I did, not exercising, doing whatever, while trying to convince myself that I was fine, that everything was fine, that I was doing great. Now that I have tasted the other side of things, I realize I was *not* fine. It was an image in my mind that I got used to. I never knew any different. This was the norm for me. Sometimes it takes someone as positive as my trainer to come into your life, to open your eyes and your mind, to allow yourself to see things from a whole different point of view.

I don't want to sound like a motivational speaker — God knows I'm not perfect, I still have a long journey ahead, one I'm sure will be full of ups and downs — but at least I'm in the right mind set. It's about keeping it there, holding onto it tightly so it doesn't crumble in my hand like a cookie, then get tossed away. I must stay focused on what I want, and on what I deserve for myself; I must put myself first instead of always last. I am just as important on this earth as anyone else.

So, on that note, once again, Happy New Year to everyone, and I hope that you, too, can reach inside yourself to make a difference in your life today, whether it be your physical self, or something completely different.

You have it in you to change, you just have to have patience, take it day by day, and know what you are doing is for the best, and that it will make YOU a stronger person. Even though what might start off as small (but positive) steps to begin with, they'll end up being the basis of the dream you might have chosen. Just strive for the best, to do your best, and in the end, it'll all work out.

Sometimes, I get ahead of myself, and my trainer has to remind me: "Step by step," and "Do what I say." What he means is *his* pace, and *he* will tell *me* when it's time for a change, whether in my exercise routine or in my diet. Patience is something I still have to get used to! Even though it seems like it takes forever, if you concentrate on what you're doing, rather than on the time it's taking, before you know it, you're there!

Friday, January 4, 2008

Two Days after Making the Front Page of the *Ottawa Sun*

I had to take a breather after seeing my picture on the FRONT PAGE of the *Ottawa Sun* newspaper. That was a shock. They never mentioned *that* part! Can you imagine? When I went to purchase a copy that morning after the gym, I was floored. "You've got to be kidding me!"

There stood a huge pile of papers with my face all over them. I started shaking. I just didn't know how to react to that. I think that shock has stayed with me until now.

Since I've had a few days to think about all this, I've been telling myself it's really important to stay on track, and not let it get to me. I can now understand how it does get to some people after having a taste of it. But I have so many other things I can't forget about, like work, kids that need to be fed and changed, swimming lessons, workouts, meetings with reporters . . . so much, I need to remember to stay focused all the time. And to remember why I am doing this first and foremost: for my health. If I make friends along the way? That's great, too.

I am very touched by the responses, the kind comments, and words of encouragement — some truly heart-warming ones. If anything, this is what's going to get me through this year, remembering that all you guys are rooting for me. I need to do this not only for myself, but for all of you, so you can all see that it's possible to change what needs to be changed. I promise you, that by the end of all this, you won't even recognize me as the same person! And yes I am *that* confident. I do not even see failure. All I see is defeat.

Saturday, January 5, 2008

Beware those Off-Days that Creep Up on You!

I think it's important, especially if you have a weight problem (or not), to understand that off-days do come along every now and again, right when you least expect them to. You have to basically tolerate them with the assurance they will pass like anything else. For me, this sort of day comes and goes once in a while. Remember to be patient, and don't give in to temptation like we all did in the past. Be stronger than IT, I guess.

It started off after I had my workout which I found really hard today. Throughout the workout, I was feeling upset and edgy which I usually don't feel (usually totally opposite). Not sure why. But one thing for sure, my trainer always hears about it!

When I got home, I just nailed him in an email with: "I think this certain exercise should change." "I find this boring." "It takes up too much time." "I don't see any use for this exercise at all."

I was just *nailing* him with complaints. (My poor trainer!) I think since we've worked together, there were only two days that he's been around to witness my attitude take a nose dive. It happened today, and about a month ago. Same thing: attitude change. But he is so sweet. Always patient and understanding. In the end, I felt kind of silly for taking out *my* negative thinking on him like I did (even though some of the stuff we discussed is true). This whole mood swing thing I'm in today didn't help, it made it seem like a bigger deal than it was.

Then there I was doing the dishes, my youngest one is crying cause she's not feeling the best (trying to be comforted by her father), my other two kids are running around the house in circles, yelling at each other and fighting. Then there's the laundry I have to tackle sometime today. And toys all over the living room floor. And I am just thinking. "*Gawd!* Take me away from here, please."

Going through my own issues, having to deal with all the extras, doesn't make it good. My tolerance level is low and I sort of go into my own . . . I don't know, my own selfish mode where I think of my own problems and try to block out everything else around me.

Plus, I have to head out to do some groceries soon. Nice. Perfect timing, wouldn't you say? I *would* say. I am SO wanting to eat the whole house at this point. And I have to face it all at the grocery store. All the wonderful smells of the bakery aisle. Seeing the chocolates . . . *hmm* . . . And all that good stuff.

On the upside, I got through this before, and I will again.

I wanted you to have a chance to understand that it isn't always as easy as people portray it to be. There are going to be days like this one, like the one I'm having right now, right at this moment! . . . but the good news is, it does pass.

I mean, while I'm writing this, I'm thinking back to two months ago, when I would have eaten. And eaten. Then when I was done, I would have felt so full and satisfied that things would have seemed better. Isn't that funny, huh? When all I was doing was storing it on my hips. Silly me. The problems and issues I was dealing with would still be there afterwards. It was pointless, now that I look back.

I take full responsibility for it all. Like I said, I took a vow never to go back to that state again, no matter how tempting it seems sometimes.

I hope you all are having a better day than I am. Stay strong people. Days like this will pass. Remember that! That's the only way I can get through them!

Thursday, January 10, 2008

I'm So Blessed

Maybe I don't have a lot of money, or a new car, or expensive clothes, or many other things people wish for, but I do have something, and that is my family, my friends, and myself! That's more than money can buy. I just *needed* something different to challenge my body and mind. Looking at what I've taken on, I think I've picked the perfect thing. There's nothing I can see myself doing, right now, that would be more challenging. (Although being who I am, it wouldn't surprise me if I think of something else once this project is finished!)

It's been a roller coaster ride! One that I'm happy I'm sharing with all of you. I wish I could reach out to each of you one by one, those who are trying to change like I am . . . to be able share these laughs together, and the stories, good, bad, happy, or sad. Laughing feels SO good! (Even when you're working your butt off. Literally!)

Friday, January 11, 2008

My Two-Month Anniversary Pictures

In eight weeks, I've already begun to transform. The changes are remarkable. As you can see, proper workouts combined with the RIGHT foods do the body good! I'm 34 pounds lighter and feelin' fantastic!

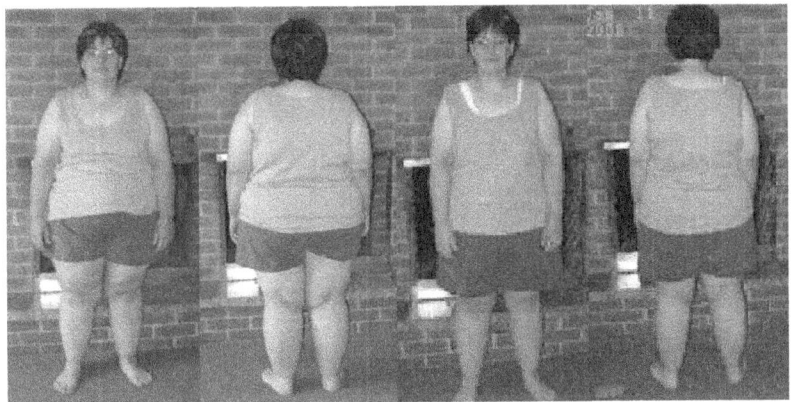

November   January

Monday, January 14, 2008

Rub-A-Dub-Dub . . . in the Tub!

Things have been going fairly well lately. I've started to drop again. My weight right now is 235 pounds, and I'm so happy about that. Five more pounds and I'll have lost 40 in just a short few months. Hard work and proper eating habits are helping me win this battle!

Something even bigger put a smile on my face this morning, another reason it's important for overweight/obese people to lose weight, another thing we all tend to miss out on without realizing it: having a bath again!

This morning I decided to have a quick bath to freshen up, and you know what? I fit so nicely in that bathtub again! I know it sounds silly, but this is the life of an overweight/obese person. It's very hard to fit in a normal bathtub, and it's not at all comfortable, either. But when I sat in it this morning, I just couldn't help admiring my legs. Even though there's still a lot of work to be done with them, they are looking much better: smaller and leaner. I thought, *I could get used to this!* I was so relaxed sitting there, I took a few extra minutes to savour the moment (along with the feeling of *Wow. I'm not squished in here anymore.*).

I suppose in the next little while, I'll be shopping at a lot of bath stores to purchase a lot of bubble bath stuff! It's something I haven't done in years. I forgot what it's like to actually relax in a bathtub. To FIT in one, comfortably!

Freedom

So again, there are so many little things we miss out on without realizing it. It's almost like a freedom others have, but one *we* don't get to enjoy. When you get it back, it feels *good!*

When you start feeling that freedom again, you start feeling as though you're in control of your own life once more. When you have no control, you just do whatever you *can* do, and shrug off what you can't. NO MORE OF THAT FOR ME! You might think about those things, and maybe decide whether or not you're going to let life pass *you* by while you accept being overweight. Do you want your freedom taken away? Or will you take charge and stand up for yourself, take the blame, and change? In the end, it's you who must make that choice. No one else! It's the best decision you'll ever make. We're all stronger than we give ourselves credit for. I'm an example of that!

When I started this transformation, I wanted to take back my life. Just this morning, I realized that's exactly what I'm doing. I'm so excited to be able to enjoy the little things again, because . . . you know what? I DESERVE IT, TOO!

Monday, January 21, 2008

40 Pounds Gone in Ten Weeks Plus a Day!

A quick note before getting my you-know-what to the gym. Today I'm feeling edgy. I don't really want to go this morning, but I know I have to. Having time away from the gym on weekends, I find Mondays always fun (NOT) to go back. But I know I'll be okay once I get there.

My weight today showed 232 pounds, so I've dropped another three since last Monday. Pretty good. I've been on this transformation for over two months and the weight drop has been steady.

I'm predicting that by March sometime, I should finally see the 100s. (*Gawd!* That is going to feel great! I haven't seen that number in so many years, I honestly can't even remember when. Once I get to 199 pounds, it will be *party time*, folks. Extra veggies for me!

I think I was about 17 when I went down to about 170–180 pounds but that was the lowest. During any diets I tried after that, the absolute lowest was 205. To think I'm almost there!

I tell you, it's going to be interesting. Not sure how I'll be at a normal weight. I can't even look that far ahead. I guess being overweight for so long will probably — no matter what — be part of my life (emotionally). I'll still sometimes see myself as that same person.

I have now passed the points of other diets that I've been on in the last few years. And once I get to that 205-pound mark (which is not that far away), I'll say to myself: *I got through that! On to the next mark at 180 pounds.* It's almost as though I have marks in my past that I'm passing by. You tend to remember a time when you were a certain weight, and what was happening in your life.

I was 180 pounds when I started dating my first boyfriend; then I was 225 pounds when I was in my last year of high school. I went up. When my brother got married ten years ago, I was able to get down to 205 pounds by working out and watching what I ate; then (I don't know what happened) back up, up, up the scale again until I reached 275 pounds which is where I started *this* whole thing.

I am never going to go back up again. All this hard work and dedication — not to mention all the wonderful things I'm learning from my trainer now, so later on, I'll know what I should or shouldn't do. I will never let myself go like I did in the past.

I have my children now. That's done with. There's no reason to gain weight. I'm sure I'll fluctuate from time to time, around 10 pounds, and I'm okay with that. But I'll be more in control of what I put into my body this time around. And I'll be the first to admit that I plan to have the Once-A-Week Pig-Out. But during the week, I'll make sure to make the most healthy choices ever. That's all. I mean I'm only normal (well . . . Italian, too!), so I still want that Once-A-Week to go eat whatever!

Altogether I've now lost 40 pounds in just over two months. Isn't that awesome? I can't believe it! I'm so proud of myself showing all of you that we can do this. See? With only patience, and hard work, and dedication, we can do anything! We do have choices.

Keep strong with me, people. Shoot out some good vibes toward me here, and any energy to give me strength. God knows, I'll need it this morning pumping those weights!

February 2008

Saturday, February 2, 2008

One of *Those* Days!

Happy weekend to you all! I'm happy it's the weekend. I'm not happy I'm having one of those I-Wish-I-Could-Eat-Everything-In-Sight Days.

It *still* happens to me sometimes. It comes creeping up when I least expect it. But it's how you choose to handle it. Doesn't help that this morning started off wrong, and I've been more on the stressed-out side today. And because I'm stressed, I want to EAT!

After all, for years, food is what I turned to to fill me up and to help me let go of, or get over, whatever was bothering me. So the thought of how good it felt eating whatever I wanted, without thinking of the consequences, still comes up and haunts me on days like today. In a sense, it was much easier back then. You *still* want to take that easy way out, sometimes. I don't think it'll ever leave me completely. You'll *always* come face to face with the option, but I refuse to take that path again.

Food was such a friend at times like this, so conveniently accessible. It would take me one second to pick up something that I shouldn't be eating and, without thinking, start eating it.

I must stay strong. I must remember that it's this same friend (food) that DESTROYED me. It took away my confidence, my energy, my right to say no, and most importantly MY LIFE! How I would just *overeat*! Lose control! I just did not have any control. But now, I'm beginning to understand the difference between "eat to live" and "live to eat." For once, I'm gaining control over foods.

From the beginning, this has been such a learning experience for me, from seeing how much I should be eating, and what foods I should be eating, to exercises that I'm becoming familiar with. All this information is vitally important so I can *stay* on this path even after I've achieved my goal. The two most important things that need balancing are PROPER food and exercise.

It's tempting, though, to take the easy way out. But when I look back at all the hard work I've been doing, at all those times when I've come face to face with choices and have been able to get *through* those times, I know I can do this!

In the meantime, to help me get over this feeling of weakness, I'm thinking good thoughts: In just nine days, it will be time for my anniversary pictures — my three-month Accomplished-And-Got-Through pictures. *That* sounds great!

I'm curious how these pictures are going to turn out in comparison to last month's, after putting my Water Theory to the test, being serious about it, making sure I'm drinking four litres a day. Will it make a big difference in the next pictures?

Time will tell.

That's also helping me keep away from eating bad things. Also, I need to weigh myself Monday to see how I did this week.

I'm just dealing with this feeling of hunger right now, but I know it will pass like everything else. (Be patient. Things will be a-okay.)

But if I should choose to give in on these weaker days . . . I know it would diminish the emotional strength I've built up during this transformation — the main thing that's going to help me down the road with any future days like this one, days which may very well end in disaster. BAD CHOICES, BAD RESULTS! I have no desire to go down *that* path. I've had such a positive outlook these last few months, it's already changed me in so many ways. I'd rather just deal with these feelings than screw up this far in the game.

Monday, February 4, 2008

Weigh-In Day!

I'm down another three pounds. I'm at 224 now. (It's still going pretty well regarding weight drops per week.) So I'm happy about that. I can almost see the 100s coming. I can't wait for that!

That's my next vision. Then there's the celebration my trainer and I will be having when I reach that point. (This will help me to keep going.) Only weeks away now when I'll finally be able to say I'm out of the 200s for GOOD!

Monday, February 11, 2008

Three-Month Anniversary Pictures!

I'm 50 pounds lighter and feeling great!

It's only been three months. I can't even imagine what my body will be like when it comes around to next January!

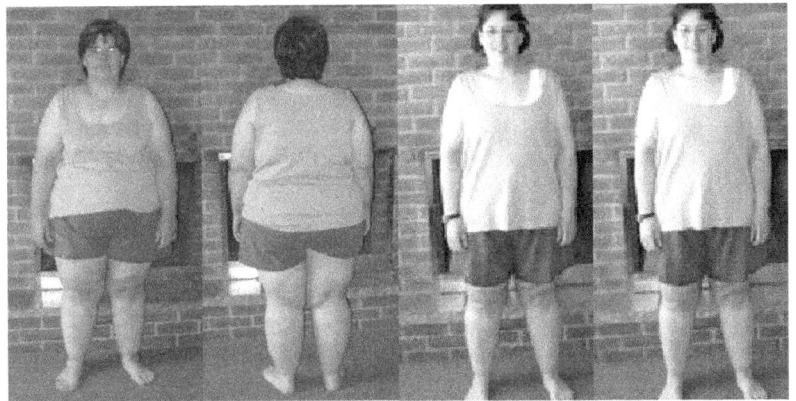

November   February

Tip of the day. Do everything in your power to NOT miss your gym days/routines. Missing gym days isn't good. When it's time to go back, it makes it that much more difficult. Even if you have time to squeeze in only 20–30 minutes, just DO IT. As few as fifteen minutes would be better than nothing. Keep the good habit going for yourself, and keep your body used to moving. Believe me, you're doing yourself a favour.

Thursday, February 14, 2008

Valentine's Day

Once again, another excuse to eat chocolates, but no chocolates for me. (*Gawd! I love chocolates.* I don't think I could ever *not* like them. Then again, I love everything, really.)

Went shopping for my little girl's Valentine cards last night after work, and I tell you, all those really nicely wrapped chocolates . . . They make them look so attractive to buy. Never mind that it's Valentine's Day! *Man!* I could barely resist. I kept looking at them, wondering what it would be like to rip one of those suckers right open and feel it melt in my mouth. Would only take half a second . . . *Yummy.* Then I snapped out of it.

I am literally counting down the days until I'm at my half-way mark. Not much more time left. Once I lose another 20 pounds, it's party time for me, kids! And party time means something really important: EATING TIME!

I have everything set in my mind, from breakfast, to lunch, to snacks, and most importantly, Chinese buffet dinner! I plan to eat a little bit of everything that day . . . because I know that is the *only* day I'll be allowed to do so until the end.

It's been tough not seeing my friends much, and not being able to do the Dinner Thing. I hope they'll all come out that night. I want to hug and kiss every one of them. I know they all understand that I'm doing something really big right now, that even though I *want* to go out, it's been tough juggling it all: work, kids, family, workouts, diet. This is the ONE night I'm looking forward to just being me, being normal like all of you! I think at this point, I surely deserve it. I'd just better watch because I might end up getting carried away and end up in the bathroom.

It will be interesting to report on how I'm feeling after that night, eating all those "bad foods" and drinking perhaps some — shall I say . . . booze? I've only had water and tea for the last three months. I'd better be *really* careful, actually!

I'll make sure to make an entry the next morning. (. . . or two mornings after, if I'm in recovery.)

Monday, February 18, 2008

Starting the Countdown!

Here's the most recent picture of me taken at the Hedley concert Saturday night. A friend took it. (We're in the bathroom — as you can tell behind me with the hand sanitizer!) But my point: Don't I look happy? This is what change does! So give it your best, people! It comes back to you a hundredfold.

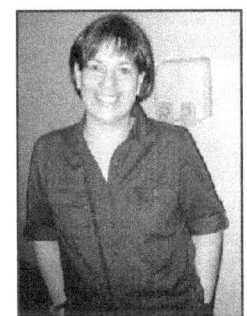

How My Friends Reacted

I had a great weekend! I had a busy Saturday, went to see one of my favourite Canadian bands, Hedley, and also saw some friends I hadn't seen in a long time. Actually, some I hadn't seen since before I even started this transformation! You can imagine how they reacted when they saw me! Let's say surprised!

Clothes Shopping for the Hedley Concert!

It felt GREAT to be able to fit into sizes 16–18! I had been in 26–28 for such a long time, the only numbers I ever saw. I got used to seeing them. Going to other racks where there are more options is a good thing.

I don't like shopping. I don't think I'll ever like shopping, but it was nice for that big change in size. I had such a hard time before. They didn't have much for me in the past, so I got used to being in jogging pants all the time.

Jogging pants were the only clothing that would be loose enough, would hide my bulge. They were convenient because they stretched! When you're big, it's all about convenience. You never want to get stressed out, so you get the quickest, easiest thing.

That life is slowly melting away. This weekend, I wore a regular pair of pants, regular top, no oversized clothes to hide anything. What people saw, was what I am. And was I ever proud!

I was glowing! Smiling a lot. I loved it. I loved being ME! For once, I felt comfortable with myself, confident, pretty again!

This has been such a journey already, and even though you do go through some downs (which I've never lied to you about because you're the first to hear about them), in the end, the up days surpass the downs. I just wish everyone could see that we all ABSOLUTELY have the power to change, if change is needed! Anyone can do it and conquer their problems. If you're reading this, and need to change something in your life that's in your way, something that's bringing you down, something that's preventing you from being the best possible person you can be (not only weight-wise but in anything), just face it, stop pushing it to the curb, stop allowing yourself to pretend that things are fine in your life when they really aren't! The best part of all this for me was admitting that I had let myself go the way I had — not only admit it to myself, but to everyone — and facing it head on and starting to fix it, one step at a time.

It was hard when I started this, to tell the world how big I was in numbers. I mean after all, it was always my greatest secret. One I held tightly so no one would *ever* know. But once I admitted it, everything was so much easier. Just because people might have certain problems, it's not the end of the world for them, although it might seem like it at the time.

When you look at life and the big picture, what are we waiting for? We all should be the best person we can be all the time. We should all be striving for that! We have the right to live a happy and healthy life, so why cheat yourself out of it? It doesn't make any sense to me why I ever let all those years pass, feeling sad inside, crying to myself some nights.

I really do wish I'd started this a long time ago, but for some reason, life wanted me to do it now, I guess. For the rest of you, there's no time like the present! Doesn't matter how old you are, or how young either. GO AHEAD AND DEFEAT IT ONCE AND FOR ALL!

Weighed myself this morning. I was so happy, I had to weigh myself maybe twenty times, and keep looking, get off, get on, look, get off, get on, look . . . That poor scale was definitely getting worked over!

TODAY'S WEIGHT IS: 216 pounds.

I'm so excited that we're in countdown mode! YES YES YES YES! 2-1-6. *2-1-6!*

I dropped 5 pounds this week alone! For a total so far of . . . 56 pounds in only three short months, plus an extra week!

I was so excited I could've peed my pants!

Thursday, February 28, 2008

This Standstill on the Scale Will NOT Get Me Down!

So . . . Woke up this morning. Okay. Couldn't help myself. Got on the scale once again, and not to my surprise, 215 pounds. *You've got to be kidding me!* I shook my head in disbelief.

After giving myself time to vent, I decided I can do one of two things: (1) let this get to me and totally be discouraged and upset and cry like a newborn baby, and freak out and shoot things around; or (2) I can go to the gym and just BLAST a weight-training workout like never before!

I chose to go with option two . . .

Once I got my daughter off on the morning school bus, I drove myself to the gym — couldn't get there fast enough — carrying with me the face of determination. I could feel it in my eyes, totally focused on getting there and giving it all I had! I refused to let a stupid scale reading get to me! No way. No how. That is not going to ruin my day, nor my views.

I blasted through my workout routine, and even upped some of the weights (one by 10 pounds!), dumbbell curls, 40 pounds. I made sure my positioning was just perfectly so, in order to give my body that perfect workout, I just pumped like there was no tomorrow. I refused to let this standstill on the scale get me down, ruin this whole transformation. I was pissed!

I had a mental picture the whole time of the body that I WILL have when I'm finished! A totally different, stronger body! The toned and muscular arms, my slimmed-down-so-completely-different-and-defined legs, my much stronger mentality! To me, this is as important as the physical aspect! It's the mental strength that will get me through maintaining my body during the many years to follow. After all, I am *not* going to lose 150 pounds to put it all back on. I DON'T THINK SO! I KNOW SO!

The thought also crossed my mind, that next December or January, I will be and will feel the healthiest ever in my life. I will be confident and smiling. I will be proud that I've overcome an obstacle that was in my way for most of my thirty-three years!

Finished the workout and was driving home . . . You know what? No matter what that scale said earlier, I felt like the strongest woman walking! I turned up that music and was so happy that I'd put in a supercharged workout!

One promise to everyone (including myself) is, that when this transformation IS over and completed, you'll see a whole different woman, one that will have the best definition. I'll be hard and strong (and headstrong!). I refuse to give up until I've reached just that!

March 2008

Sunday, March 2, 2008

The Countdown Continues . . . Will It Stay?

I've decided to start going to the gym first thing in the morning again to do my cardio, which is where I just got back from. It gets my day off on the right foot, and I love starting my day off right!

Later this morning, I'll be back at my "other" gym, Free Form Fitness, to do my weight-training session before heading off to work. The three days a week when I weight train are going to be tougher because I've decided to do five days a week of cardio instead of just the two. But no matter what, I still have a personal responsibility to include my weight training — as an extra — during three of those days! Am I crazy? Maybe. But I feel I can do it, so why not try? I like to push and challenge myself now, whenever I can. So this morning was the first of many mornings. This will be a bonus for my trainer to see how this works with someone while weight training. It may turn out great, or I may burn myself out. Time will tell, I suppose.

I'm not going to get all my hopes up, but the scale this morning read 211 pounds, now 64 pounds lost in total — just in case you don't remember that I started at 275. If everything goes well, hopefully the numbers will continue to go down in the next few weeks.

I suppose I'm already somewhat hooked on this new lifestyle. The cardio part gets me full of energy, and that gets me through my day. The weight training makes me feel strong as I build muscle. And the eating? Well, I'm only eating Nature's best, which is helping with the output

my body is showing me which is everything—
from my hair, to my skin — my whole body! It's
been fantastic in that sense.

Sunday, March 9, 2008

Weight Is Not the Only Thing I've Lost!

Sunday night and I feel like writing. I'll be on
tomorrow to reveal my weight, but tonight I have
something else I want to share: I lost something
else Friday afternoon — my engagement ring!

Yes, pretty sad. Not sure where, but I think
somewhere at work. It must have slipped right off
my hand without my noticing (nor feeling, nor
hearing it as it fell).

So I've been kind of in the dumps about that. I've
worn that ring since before my husband and I got
married (about six and a half years), never took it
off. I continued wearing it as we built our life, and
as the children followed.

This weekend, I feel I'm missing something. I
can't help thinking about it. It obviously shows
that even my fingers are getting smaller, but I'm
pretty down about it.

Rings like that have a story to them. All I can say
is, it really sucks! It was a setting that went with
my wedding band.

Anyway. Just giving you a warning. If you plan to
lose lots of weight . . . I guess after the 50-pound
mark, take the rings off!

Monday, March 10, 2008

. . . and My Weight Is . . .

208 pounds.

67-pound loss in total.

So I dropped a few more as of last Monday. It's slowly going down. It's funny, but now that I'm in the countdown stages to the 100s, it seems to be taking a long time . . . however, I tend to forget how far I've come along!

Another 9 pounds and I'll be there. It cannot come FAST enough!

Great News! What Was Once Lost Has Been Found!

I found my ring! Well, actually a co-worker did.

And . . . not to anyone's surprise, I'll NOT be wearing it anymore until the end of this transformation project when I'll then resize them both!

I've learned my lesson!

Tuesday, March 11, 2008

Four-Month Anniversary Photos

These are just the start of what's going to be happening as we go along. Once the actual weight is taken off, then you'll be the first to see the sculpting, and some bodybuilding as well. I'm *so* excited!

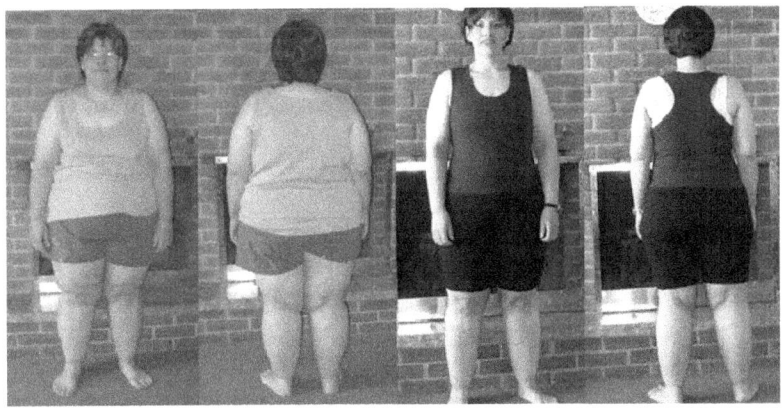

November   March

Saturday, March 15, 2008

Changes Happen from Head to Toe When You Choose to be Healthy

This close up picture of me was taken this afternoon.

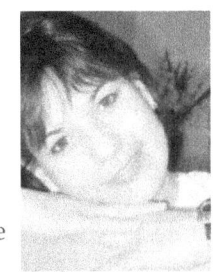

Some people have been saying lately that I'm starting to look younger since losing this weight? Hmm . . . You can be the judge. Look at my first picture and compare. You'll notice that my face *does* look a lot different (and no I'm not talking about the obvious, that the older one looks fuller). Look at my eyes in this picture, how bright they are, my skin's clear; even my hair looks healthy! There's just a natural glow about me, such a happier look.

When you make a change to nourish your body with the right HEALTHY foods, instead of eating all that junk out there (that we're all addicted to in some way), it'll make a huge difference in the way your outside will look. For me: four months — that's 16 weeks! — of eating purely natural, NOTHING other than good-for-me foods, lots of water, workouts five days a week . . . and this has been the result. So far! Imagine later on!

Healthy foods are all I know now. This comes when all you do is eat right, day after day. It's something you learn and something that becomes the norm! It's like your thoughts on foods just get reversed and reset your brain.

As time goes on, resisting those foods helps you become strong, and you don't need nor want those foods anymore. As you get used to working out every day, that too becomes a whole new healthy habit. It makes you feel so great afterwards! Now that I think about it, I'm not sure if I'm addicted to working out, or if I'm addicted to the feeling I get after my workouts. It's a natural high!

It was hard in the beginning to go without any cheat days. I can't lie to you about that. To not even have one bite of anything was torture for the first little while. But believe it or not, it got easier and easier as time went on, until I got to the point where it didn't bother me at *all!* It hasn't bothered me since!

If you find yourself in the same boat I was in, and would like to break free from this addiction to bad eating habits, the best way to tackle this problem is to just NOT HAVE ANY OF THEM. I cannot stress that point enough: act as though those sorts of foods no longer exist! This is what saved me!

Obviously, my trainer knew what he was doing — although at the time I didn't understand why he was so strict, why it was that I couldn't have that one day a week to cheat like on other so-called diets. It's obvious to me now.

It's funny because I *love* the SMELL of bad foods these days. I always want to smell them and I don't really know why. Even though I have no real desire for them, if someone is eating them, when the smell comes around, I just want to take a moment to smell! The great thing is, there are no calories in the pleasure of smelling.

Monday, March 17, 2008

The Countdown Continues!

Back from the gym. This morning's weigh-in showed 204 pounds, so that's now a total of 71 pounds to date. *Yes!*

I'm pretty happy about that! At this moment, I have nothing to complain about. Things are going according to plan, and I'm pretty sure I can lose another 6 pounds by April 18 when we have our half-way-mark party. (Most probably before, unless I hit some kind of crazy, annoying badly timed plateau.)

Monday, March 24, 2008

An Apple A Day Keeps the Doctor Away

Before going to the gym for my cardio this morning, I jumped on that scale of mine and when I looked at the numbers (205 pounds), I should have been really upset, but I wasn't.

I started my new diet yesterday (Sunday). It's more like the first diet I was on. I'm more than confident that the numbers are going to start dropping again, this time probably more consistently. So nothing to be upset over. After all, this is a lifetime change I'm doing! So what if we are playing around a little bit. We're learning as we go about this great body of mine, and what it wants — *needs* — to work to its full potential. Even though I don't remember offhand what yesterday's inches lost were, I do know they were pretty crazy.

Imagine

Imagine you were really heavy all your life, and in just over four months, you dropped 70 pounds, along with tons of inches. You start feeling things you never used to feel, noticing and seeing certain bones you never knew were even there, and your face is slimming right down. It's been so rapid, it's crazy but amazing at the same time.

I'm witnessing first hand what's been hiding underneath all the extra skin I carried around for so long. It's like a new person is starting to come out. It's not only physical things I notice, but me as a person. Sometimes it's overwhelming.

All my life, I just got way too comfortable with the fact that I was overweight, and in my mind I always thought *This is what I am. This is what I'll always be.* I was taught to accept it!

(It was much easier to accept my weight issue than actually *do* something about it. When I *did* get up the courage to try to change, I faced the reality that I had a lot of work ahead of me. This, in turn, discouraged me, so I would fail.)

I lived it for most of my life, so all these changes I'm going through during this transformation shock even me most times.

Sunday, March 30, 2008

Starting to Love to Shop! Surprises Always Await

Looking at myself in the mirror now when I go shopping these days, I can't believe the person who stares back at me.

What really impresses me? My *arms!* The same arms I've been working out on for the past five months have changed big time. Even without flexing I can see the definition, the muscles developing there. *Oh, boy!* First thought? *Where's my trainer, damn it?* It was so exciting to see. These days, when people feel my arms, they're always harder there. Crazy, crazy stuff! Unbelievable how my body is constantly changing from one stage to another.

Remember? Before I made the decision to change, I believed the fat life, the obese life was what *my* life was supposed to be. Now? I was so wrong. If you're reading this, and you're overweight, or obese . . . *You are* so wrong *as well!* It can be done!

This is what I'm so happy to show you all. I'm taking you through this journey alongside me, from one extreme to another. We all have the ability to do this! It's about taking charge, making a decision, and sticking with it even through the tough days. You'll have days like last night, when you find yourself being amazed and excited for tomorrow, full of smiles, and laughter, and confidence. It's great. It makes all the hard work and determination worth it. Worth all of it!

My life is in the hands of my trainer now, and I just do what he asks when it comes to eating, when it comes to exercises (even when the exercises seem silly to me . . .). It's been really amazing so far. I realize now he chooses them all for a reason.

Very proud moment for me!

We'll need a drum role for Monday.

Monday, March 31, 2008

Another Weigh-In Day

Well, this morning before heading off to the gym for my cardio, I weighed myself, which is my duty to you guys . . . Looking down I saw 201 pounds.

201?

I really thought this Monday I would be either 200 pounds, or even out of the 200s. It looks like I'll probably have to live with being still in the 200s for one more week. (I hope that's all.)

But it hasn't really got me down. I'm just trying to keep my head up and think *Oh well. It's just a scale.*

Plus! . . . I've now hit the 74 pounds in total weight loss since starting, so basically there's only 1 more pound to lose before I can actually say I'm halfway to my end goal. THAT is something to be *happy* about.

But . . . let's hope for a more impressive number on the scale next time around!

April 2008

Monday, April 7, 2008

I'm Now in the 100s Category!

Yay! Yes. It is most certainly true!

I've not only hit my half-way mark in this transformation project, but I've surpassed it!

My weight now, as of the reading from this morning, is 197 pounds! That's right! One hundred and ninety-seven pounds!

Gawd that feels GREAT to be able to say that finally! Just an incredible feeling!

I've been in the two hundreds for probably seventeen years. What a rush! So . . . Total weight loss to date is now 78 pounds! This means my trainer and I are pretty much right on schedule.

Wednesday, April 9, 2008

I Hate How I'm Feeling Today

I was disappointed watching the playback of myself on TV on the Rogers "Daytime" show. I don't like myself on camera at *all!* I can't wait for the day when I see myself on Rogers "Daytime" show and can say "Hey. I don't look too bad."

For now, I'm not enthused about it. I hated my hair, so I cut it myself this morning. Gave myself a little trim on the sides. That's me — when I want to do something I just do it . . . without thinking. My hair didn't turn out too badly given that I'm not a hairdresser. I felt better after I cut it. I don't know . . . I guess how I looked got me upset and I took it out on my hair.

Even though I lost 78 pounds, I still go through crappy days when I see myself and think I look terrible. It doesn't matter how many people tell me otherwise, some days are just harder.

Watching myself sitting there on the program (if I may be honest), I thought I looked huge! I thought I looked much bigger than in person. My stomach had rolls and I just looked gross. Anyway . . . There you have it. The pure honesty of it all.

I was disappointed! I went in there feeling so confident, and then watching later, was shocked, upset. But I'm not as sad now that I've had time to sleep on it because I know I'll continue to get closer to my goal and won't be looking at myself like that. After all, there won't be much left TO me in the end.

Thought I'd write about it nevertheless. It's important to share both the good and the BAD. And this is one of the bad.

Five-month pictures coming up on the 11th. Hold onto your seats. Slowly, we are getting there.

Missing My Friends

I saw a friend the other day. He came over for business-related stuff. I had missed him so much, I gave him the biggest hug! I never realized how hugs feel so great during times like these, how you really appreciate your friendships even more!

I suppose seeing *him* made me miss *all* my friends whom I don't get to see as much as I'd like to.

Having kids plus work, taking on this project has been like another job in a way. And I'm having to fit it all in. But we all do what we have to do. I know my true friends understand. I guess it hit me when I saw him: how I miss those days when I could just go out and have whatever, do whatever, and not always be thinking and thinking, and making choices.

I know this project is not forever, but I'm telling you it's been hard. Yes, I've gotten stronger, but it's tough to change so drastically in such a short time. Your emotions are sometimes all over the place. I know I'll get there soon enough . . . but you have these emotional days where it just hits you so hard.

Later . . .
What a nice surprise when I got home from work!

When I got back from work, one of my best friends, Elena, had surprised me by having flowers delivered, congratulating me on reaching the half-way mark. They could not have come at a better time. I hadn't received flowers in about two years, so it put a smile on my face.

Thanks so much! I needed that.

Thursday, April 10, 2008

The Emotional Weight-Loss Roller Coaster Continues . . .

Here are few things I need to write about to give you an example of the ups and downs of a journey like this.

Yesterday was a real down . . . worst down I've had in a while.

But I got through it. I went to my workout today.

I also went shopping after work. I have to tell you that I ran into an Italian couple I haven't seen in a while. They didn't even recognize me! Can you believe that? I was stunned. They got into the questions: "My godda how you loose so mucha weight? You no get sick eh?"

"No!" I replied with (of course) the biggest smile ever. "I work out hard," I told them. "And I eat well now."

They were in shock, I guess.

(Italians seem always to assume, when someone loses weight, it's because they are sick, or will get sick. One of the two.)

After that encounter, I had to use the bank machine. (I also had to do a quick run to the bathroom because of the water I've started drinking again.)

While there, I thought I'd take a moment to check out a few stores because I really needed to do some shopping for a few events coming up.

Walking by a plus-size store, I glanced at it and just kept walking (hard to believe I don't have a place in that store anymore). Then for the FIRST TIME, I walked right across to the regular-size store instead. *Man.* That was WEIRD! While in there (basically taking a glimpse around to see what that store carries), I thought to myself: *Anytime now, someone is going to approach me and tell me that the plus store is across the way.* I almost felt strange and out of place to be there. It was the weirdest feeling! In a sense, it was almost hard to believe I was actually in there. In just nineteen weeks, I've changed this much? *Wow.*

But no one said anything.

Then I thought, *I'm going to try this again.* (At this point, it was almost like having a cheap thrill!) This time, it was the new store around the corner! I always thought they had nice clothes, but never even bothered going in there ever because I always knew I wouldn't fit into anything.

Well, I walked in and looked around. I have to say they had *nice* stuff! Then I thought, *What the hell,* and grabbed a few pants that looked really nice. Size 16, of course. And off I went to try them on. (I had only a few minutes to do this because Mom was watching the kids, and waiting for me to get home from work.)

They fit! And they fit well! Some not as perfectly as I would have wanted, but only because of style. But they fit! It was like being reassured that *Yes, I am a size 16.* It's not some dream I'm dreaming up. One pair was actually a little big. Going from a size 26–28 to a 16? *Wow!* My trainer must really know what he's doing regarding food and exercise. I'm a perfect example of that! We have definitely proved to everyone what everyone already knew about him. He KNOWS HIS STUFF.

When I came out of that change room? *Boy!* Was I sporting the biggest smile ever! I stood there and took another glance around the store, thinking *Oh my gawd! Now I can pick out any one of these outfits! I can choose any different style now if I like, and I know they'll have my size! No more taking only what I can get. I have a huge assortment to choose from now!*

The lady approached me while I was thinking about all this in my head. And smiling. She asked if there was anything else she could help me with.

I replied: "No. I really have to go. But I'll *definitely* be back soon!" I was thinking that my eyes were so big and excited, she probably thought I was high on drugs or something. When I walked out of there, I felt like a million bucks!

Friday, April 11, 2008

Five-Month Anniversary Pictures

One hundred and ninety-six pounds.

Here they are. I've included the originals from November 11, and the rest are: my front and back, and some fun pictures for you to enjoy.

I've come along quite a bit in just twenty weeks. Still a lot to do, but it's coming.

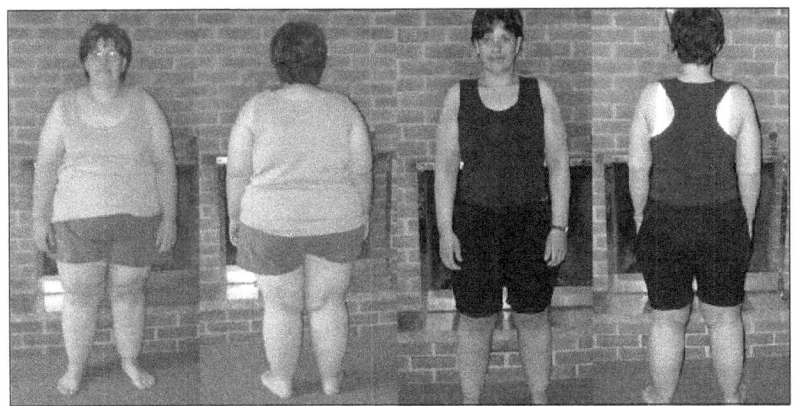

November   April

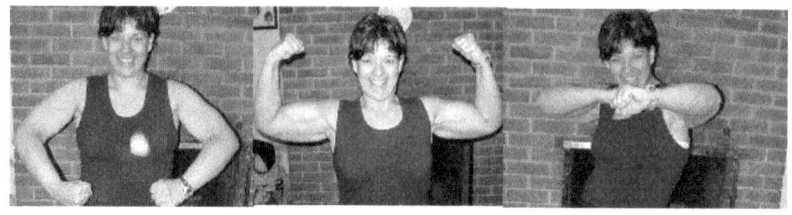

Monday, April 14, 2008

Four Days until Our Party

What a morning it's starting out to be!

First things first: my weigh-in today! I got on the scale and I've dropped some pounds once again over the weekend! Must have been that extra dancing I did. Busta moving on the dance floor on Saturday.

I'm now 194 pounds! That's right. I usually do best out of three, but all three times said the same thing, so I've now lost a total of 81 pounds! I'm excited because the next leap is soon approaching — to have lost 100 pounds! *Oh my gawd.* To write that is going to be something else!

How do I feel right now? I feel wonderful! I feel more confident, energized, ready to take on the world and whatever it brings! It also helped that today I brought along an MP3 player with some really pumpin' sounds for the gym. Imagine me driving to the gym this morning at 6:00 a.m., just pumpin' that music, ready to really kick it this week! It was awesome! At the gym, it actually helped a lot. I don't even know how I went on for five months with no music at all, only watching soundless TV at the gym, while listening to people (including me) breathing hard.

Never too late to start the MP3 era. (I feel old and out of the loop when it comes to technical things. I never knew you could hook one of those up to the stereo in the car! Awesome stuff, this feeling young again.)

This week, I plan to give it all I've got until Friday. I'll be getting ready for our half-way-mark party that I'm so excited about. (I've been counting down to this party for months!)

Reasons why I'm excited: (1) I'll see all my friends again. I haven't seen them in so long. And I miss them! I have tons of hugs to go around that night, so believe me, it's going to be a love-fest! (2) I'll meet all the new friends who've been following our story. That's exciting! (3) I'll be able to eat some really bad stuff on the Saturday! (Saturday is the ONLY day my trainer, Rob, says I can do this food part.)

I have it all planned out . . . (I chose to eat Saturday by the way, so if my body reacts badly, it will happen at home, and not at the party while meeting people. That wouldn't be smart.)

So I'm making my list of foods starting with walking into a store and actually buying a chocolate bar (weird); and then some liquorice; and chips; and nachos; and Chinese buffet! Whatever I want! Oh. And I'll need to have some alcoholic drinks on Friday for my party night, too. Better mark that down on the list!

Now, I'm not sure how my body is going to react to all that really bad man-made greasy stuff, sweets, and drinks, et cetera. I might even end up going back to having cravings again. Not really sure *how* it will affect me physically and emotionally — probably clog my stomach (or opposite!), or make me bust out in massive pimples. I don't know. But after five months of not eating or drinking anything bad for me, it should be an interesting experiment, so I'm going to go for it! You can read how I feel afterwards. It will be something, to see how my body reacts to "bad" stuff, because this is what we as a society in general, are eating. It's how I used to eat all the time. It will show me (and us) what most of us put into our bodies on a daily basis. Perhaps it's killing us!

You can all look forward to how I feel after this weekend, after drinking (alcohol) and eating like old times. I might turn out to be really sick. I have no idea. I will be stepping into new not-so-good territory. But it will be fun to read about it later.

Saturday, April 19, 2008

My Cheat-Day Menu

Okay. Here I am. Alive, but barely.

First, the party. It was nice. It was fun. I didn't drink much, only one glass of wine and half a beer. That's it. I didn't need any more. That wine hit me pretty hard. But all in all, I saw many friends I had not seen since starting this project and that was the nicest part of the whole night.

Today was my actual Cheat Day for eating. I picked up my trainer, Rob, and we started our eating about 1:00 in the afternoon and didn't finish until 4:00 p.m. But it didn't end there. That night, I went for the buffet (Chinese), and now, I'm finishing off my Cheat Day with a Big Mac and medium fries — but barely getting through it.

So while I'm slowly (and I mean *slowly*) eating my last bad meal, I decided to write at the same time.

As far as food today? Absolutely *nothing* healthy went into my mouth at all. Totally opposite from what I've been taught the last five months. What did I eat, you may ask?

Well . . .

Breakfast: four slices of toast with margarine *and* peanut butter on all of them. About four glasses of milk to make it go down smooth.

I tried a Doritos chip later that morning thinking I was going to enjoy it, but could only eat one because it tasted as though I'd put a tablespoon of salt into my mouth. (No chip flavour there like the ones I remembered. Perhaps it was because I ate them all the time?)

Then, as I mentioned above, I picked up Rob for lunch and we started by eating at one of my favourite restaurants: restaurant nachos topped with melted cheese, sauce, green onions, olives, and I must not forget the sour cream on the side for dipping. We also got a combination platter with that, which included deep-fried zucchini, honey garlic wings, and potato skins. (We decided to stick with water which is probably the only decent thing we did today.)

After that lunch, we walked around a little, and stopped at a store in the mall where we purchased a pack of fresh red liquorice, and a pack of Ferrero Rocher chocolates.

While eating the Ferrero Rocher chocolates, we drove to a Dairy Queen for a treat. I had a medium vanilla cone, and Rob had a medium dipped in chocolate.

When we were done, we got back into the car and continued driving until we stopped somewhere else to take a break, only to get back into the car where we opened the bag of liquorice to start eating that on the way home. (I ate quite a few of those, perhaps 10 pieces.)

My day of cheating did not end there. No sir! For supper I went to the Chinese buffet where I ate: chicken fried rice, chicken balls, onion rings, egg rolls, soup (forget the name), some garlic spare ribs, and . . . I think that was it. Oh. I can't forget the sauces on top. (We also had cake and more ice cream there. And a fortune cookie.)

Later, when I came home, I had another cookie.

. . . and now, I'm attempting to finish that Big Mac and medium fries I told you about . . . but looking at it . . . I'm only half way through . . . I don't think I can finish it . . .

So there you have it. A full day of nothing but the worst things. And all in one day.

How do I feel?

My stomach obviously has grown a few inches to say the least, and I feel really bloated, tired, and it's as if the food is just sitting there and has not moved. Mostly ALL the stuff I ate today . . .

I have to say the one ingredient that stood out the very most was that taste of salt in my mouth. Foods never seemed salty to me in the past. It seems like almost all have a high content of salt.

My tongue feels weird, as if I burned it eating the foods (and I've been really thirsty).

At the Chinese buffet, even though my foods ended up being just one-plate-and-a-half worth, I had to get up and go outside because I felt so full. I almost felt anxious because I just couldn't sit there. My heart was beating faster. Once I got some air and stood outside for a while, I felt a bit better, so I went in, paid the bill, and went home.

One thing!
Tomorrow. I cannot *wait* to eat my own food again. I don't like the way I feel tonight. I'm not down about what I ate at all — I mean it's one day — but physically I feel so big right now, so heavy, and I'm still glancing over at the McDonald's thing, and honestly, I can't finish it.

Believe me, I tried really hard.

But it's now 11:12, so I have less than an hour left before this Cheat Day is over. Then I'll not be allowed to eat any of these foods again, pretty much until the end. (At this point, I can truthfully say I don't have a problem with that!)

My eyes feel heavy. I'm ready to sleep, but there's no way I can lie down with this stomach of mine.

Anyway. That was my Cheat Day. If anything changes, I will write again tomorrow, or in the next few days. Right now, I think I need to walk a little, and throw out the rest of this McDonald's.

I'll still weigh myself on Monday. Also, don't forget I was 194. We'll see what I am on Monday, how my body reacted to all this food.

Monday, April 21, 2008

Weigh-In Day. Up 2 Pounds

Yesterday, I have to say, I was getting cramps in my stomach all day, but other than that, the really bad food didn't hurt me too much. However, I was beat! I was so tired I had to take a nap, something I haven't done in months. My energy was low, hardly energy enough to do laundry. It was insane.

But, this morning I was back to normal. I headed off to burn all those extra calories I'd gained on Saturday. This morning, I was surprised that my energy was actually pretty high during my cardio.

The downfall was when I went to weigh myself this morning. Looks like I gained 2 pounds! I went up to 196. But it could have been worse. At least I'm not in the 200s anymore. After all, it's only numbers. Nothing my cardio and weight training won't get rid of this week. (I hope.)

Thursday, April 24, 2008

The Smell of Summer Is in the Air!

Lately I've been feeling really good. Although for a few days after eating all that "bad" stuff with my trainer, my energy level was really, really low. Not sure why, not even sure if the actual foods had anything to do with it. But it seems it has now passed and I'm back up to par energy-wise.

Since Monday, I've noticed I'm sweating a lot more during cardio. I believe it's a good thing. The more I sweat, the more I'm losing. All in all I've been feeling just terrific these days.

Friday, I'm meeting with my trainer, Rob Lagana, to up my routine again. He's excited to show me this routine and tells me I'm going to love it. (But when Rob says that, I know the chances are it's going to kill me for the first few weeks!)

April is soon coming to an end, so I'm getting ready to crack out some shorts and tanks this summer. I cannot wait for that! To be able to wear those things, and feel great, is going to be something really different for me. Year after year, I wore long pants (half the time they were heavy joggers), but NO MORE, I SAY! This summer is MY summer and I'm taking back MY right to be normal, to be able to wear things I like.

But . . . This transformation is not going to take too much longer. I'm hoping that by the time November rolls around (when it will be exactly one year since I started) I'll be there at the end, and finished.

Since I missed last year's Christmas time, it would be nice to sit down and enjoy a really great supper. We all have to do what we have to do to get what we want in life . . . I've missed a lot, but I've gained much more by missing those things — if that makes sense.

I look back and I cannot believe how I, and many millions of people, live day by day, every day, merely accepting how we are, instead of taking responsibility, facing up to our flaws, and just changing. It makes you a stronger person inside and out, really! There's nothing negative that comes out of something like this. It's all positive and makes you a better person.

I know it's difficult to make a commitment to change, and to keep at it, but you know, it doesn't take all that long to get to the goal if you actually stick with it! It seems like it does, but for me, I can't believe it's been almost six months. And I'm still going strong! I suppose I was ready for it this time around. Ready to give it all I had, the one last hope that I could do this.

Now, I can start reaping the rewards of my hard work by finally having the freedom I never had, the confidence I never carried, and a real sense of what happiness is all about.

We all can have that, you know. For those reading this and thinking "Oh. Good for her. But I'm just stuck," OPEN YOUR EYES! YOU'RE NOT STUCK AND WERE NEVER STUCK! This is your laziness speaking for you. Or, better yet, you've accepted being how you are now, just like I used to. But WHY? Why accept it?

You can change starting today. But there's only one person who can make that decision. And that's you! No one can make it for you, and believe me, I know. If you're not ready to change, you won't.

It's funny, because YOU just know inside when you're TRULY ready to make a change. It's a certain feeling, different from the other trials and failures. It's a feeling of readiness to accept all that's difficult. You have a picture in your head of working hard, sweating tears — missing your foods — but at the same time you think, *Well? This is how it's going to be and I'll do what I have to do!* You leave behind the excuses you once had and start from scratch. It becomes a new way of life for you after a while. You still bitch and complain at times, and have bad days, but your heart is always striving for the end goal.

Monday, April 28, 2008

Monday Weigh-In

Four pounds down with only 67 pounds to go until I finish this project!

Since last Monday, I've lost another 4 pounds (I'm standing at 192 pounds), so that pig-out I had last week didn't really affect me much.

Last Monday I only went up 2 pounds (surprised myself after all the food I ingested!), but it's all good. Back down again now, minus another 2!

Things are pretty much back on track! I don't foresee anything coming up in the near future, which could set me back — other than the BIGGEST piece of cake for the next celebration. (However, the way my body's been performing lately, I'm sure it will just eat it up in no time!)

The celebration I'm talking about of course, will be reaching the 100-pound-total-weight-loss point! This is what I'm now trying to put all my focus on, reaching that next goal. It will be a BIG (probably the biggest) milestone for me! And I'm very close to reaching it now! Only 17 pounds left until I hit that mark!

What's 17 pounds? Not much considering the weight I've lost already, or the ups and downs I've gone through over the past (almost) six months to get here. So bring it on, I say!

Things in general have been going well, although last week, I had the odd day when I was very tired. People have been sick around me, but I don't really get sick anymore. (Weird, eh?) Physically, I've been feeling tired. Maybe that's how my body is handling a sickness instead of getting it full force. I don't know.

It's surprising because I'm never tired anymore, I haven't needed to take naps since I started this project. (By the way, this is the up-side to changing your lifestyle to a more active one. You have much more energy.) So for me to be tired is a strange thing. Oh well, I'm sure it will pass!

I have to run. I'm late. (Nothing new.) I'm tackling my new workout today, then have to get to work afterwards.

May 2008

Sunday, May 11, 2008

Six-Month Anniversary Pictures! Half Way There . . .

When I started this project back in November, I made a vow, a promise, to give it everything I had while I attempted to lose 150 pounds in one year! It would have to be done naturally, without pills or fad diets, or surgery. Some thought I'd fail, others thought I wouldn't last, but here I am, six months later and still going strong!

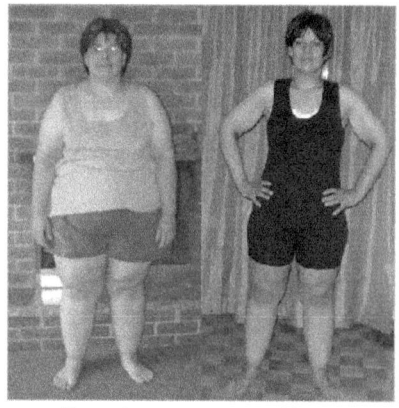

November   May

Monday, May 12, 2008

Being a Kid Again

Let's get right to the point. Weigh-in showed 187 this morning. and at first I was a little disappointed with that number, but hey, two pounds is better than no pounds at all!

So 88 pounds of total weight loss in six months! Wow! I see that 100-pound mark approaching!

For the First Time . . .

Obviously, I and a lot of mothers out there celebrated Mother's Day over the weekend. For the first time, I really, really enjoyed my Mother's Day. My sister and I took the kids to the Experimental Farm. (They had a special thing for Mother's Day, cheaper prices, too.) There was a play structure there, and it was such a great feeling to go up those stairs with my littlest one, Emma, who's almost two, and not have to turn to the side to go up those stairs! (They are made fairly small. In the past, I would have to go up them sideways.) So I was happy about that. Felt fantastic holding her hand while climbing. Something even better: Once I would get to the top (I rarely went, for this reason), I would go back down to let the kids go down themselves, because I always thought I was too big for the slide. WELL! Not *this* time! Down I went with my little one. She just looked at me. I think she, too, was surprised. I was so excited, we went up them quite a few times. It was so much fun! I really missed out on that in the past. It's fun being a kid again, not worrying about people looking at you, and wondering what they're saying. It's the best feeling in the world!

One other thing about my littlest one: Over the weekend, I gave her a bath and I got into the tub with her! I was never able to do that. It was great! It puts a smile on my face just thinking about it. I was able to bathe her, and play with her, with her toys, and I FIT! Comfortably. With lots of extra room left. Amazing!

These are only a few of the great things I can now enjoy. This weekend, I had a taste of what it's really like to play with your kids, to enjoy them, and cherish them. When you feel good, it makes such a difference — even in the lives of your children. They see it, they feel it . . . and that's what it's all about.

Man! Over the weekend, I saw a glimpse of what life will finally start being like from now on. It's as though a big weight has been lifted off you. You can breathe again, you can have your freedom back, you can play with your kids and not be such a grump. Or, not have to stay home like I did in the past because mentally I was just not there. I have a lot of making up to do with my kids and that's exactly what I plan to do!

For me, my weight held me back from a lot of things throughout my life, and this is really what losing weight is all about. It's not about numbers on the scale, it's not about boasting. You have to look deep down inside yourself when you're ready to change your life the way I chose to, and to really have those reasons — good *real* reasons why you're doing it because that is what will take you right through. Anything superficial, and you'll fail, or it won't last.

This is something I actually recall talking about with my trainer, Rob, when he first came over to do my original assessment. He told me to really think about *why* I wanted to lose weight. He told me flat out: "If the reasons are on a superficial level, you won't make it. They have to be real true reasons, so that, when you're having those bad days, you'll be able to remember those reasons and will continue to succeed because they'll mean a lot to you."

My kids *do* mean a lot to me. They are my world. To be able to share this life with them in a healthier, more fun way? I'm overjoyed by that!

Rosy's Top Five Tips to Help You Stay on Track

(1) Have a mental picture in your mind, and PLAN your weight-loss project.

Any successful project starts with a plan, and you need to look at losing weight the same way. Think about where you stand presently, where you want to be, and the steps you'll take to get there! Plan your meals and prepare them in advance. This has helped me tremendously!

(2) Look at your weight loss project as a life-changing experience. Not as a diet.

Focus more on the idea that you have now chosen and made a commitment to take the path of a healthier lifestyle. You'll start to witness your body change and become new. Start by promising yourself to allow nothing but healthy foods in, to watch your portion control, and to start to take small steps to make exercise part of your new daily lifestyle. Join a gym if you can, and if money is an issue for you, there's always the local YMCAs which have a program in place to help with funds because *everyone* deserves to live a healthier active life!

(3) Use all the resources you can to help make this project succeed.

Visit your local library, do some online searches, talk to your family doctor. Get EXCITED about re-educating yourself on how you can change your unhealthy body into a brand new healthier one! You'll be surprised at how much information is out there, and how amazing this sort of project becomes! Just remember: nothing will be handed to you, it's up to you to take charge of your own life, and to act on it!

(4) Get mentally prepared by acknowledging the fact that it's not going to be easy.

This might be the BIGGEST challenge you'll ever take, but remember, the rewards to oneself which come from being challenged are 100 times better. Being challenged makes you a stronger person both inside and out. Also remember to keep in mind — especially if you're having a bad day — in the end, it *will* be all worth it, and it certainly *does* get easier as times goes on. Stay strong, don't let weakness defeat you, you're much stronger than that. Have patience, work through it day by day, week by week. Don't focus on the end goal.

(5) Set little goals before reaching your end goal.

This will make the time go by faster, and you'll be excited when passing these little goals as you reach them. You won't even realize you're getting closer to the bigger goal with each passing day. These can be anything from special monthly occasions, weekly weigh-ins, monthly pictures. Perhaps your doctor can arrange some weekly weigh-ins, FREE OF CHARGE! Do whatever you can that'll help keep you motivated while you work toward your end goal.

We all deserve to be healthier and happier, so challenge yourself today!

Friday, May 16, 2008

Trying to Get through a Tough Day

Thought I'd write about my day today because it's important to me that everyone experience my harder days as well as my easy ones, so they'll know it's normal to go through them, and that mentally we *can* get through them.

I was so hungry today! More than usual. Not sure if it was due to cravings or if I actually *was* hungry. I don't know what's been going on lately. My cravings have altered more than usual, and especially today, they were really high. I was at work, and there was a box of Tim Horton's Timbits sitting right there in the staff room. *Man!* I could just taste those things. Nice and fresh and sweet and just plain ol' yummy. It took everything in me to not go over there and eat the whole box.

Lately it's been hard because I've been craving sweets a lot. Especially cake.

It's like you're fighting a battle in your head when that happens. You're debating and thinking, continuously going back and forth with yourself.

At one point I thought *I could have just one.* Then I thought *No I can't.* Then I thought *I'm going to a wedding tomorrow. It probably won't be so bad if I had some sweets there for tomorrow.* Then again *No I can't.* And then *Oh my god, there's still six months to go of this. I'm going to die. I'm really going to die! No I won't.*

I moped around a little with a really blah face on me, feeling sorry for myself that I cannot be like

117

other people enjoying those sweets (which I am sure taste so friggin' good in their mouths). Then at one point I found myself looking in the mirror at work, and thinking, *Wow. I look slim today.* (Probably my mind trying to make the whole ordeal into a positive thing.) . . . but then I would come back saying. "I have to talk to my trainer because my arms are looking flabby." IT WAS INSANE TODAY!

That is what my day was like . . . in my own little world, having lots of conversations with myself. But bottom line is, it's all about staying strong. If you don't give in, you'll be okay. Really. But in the meantime, it's just plain ol' tough and seems like the hardest thing to get through!

I still have a lot of weight to get off and, to be honest, I'd rather suffer for another six months to get it done and over with, than have the odd cheat that could potentially set me back big time, or even destroy what I've accomplished so far!

It's going to be nice later on, once I've reached my goal, to be able to go to the gym three times a week, and to eat healthy during the week, then to splurge one day on the weekend or at the odd occasion that comes up. But right now, it would not do me any good to do that.

Thinking about it, though, I'm wondering if this has all come on because I've been feeling down about not losing much these last few weeks. Perhaps more down than I've let on to others (or to myself). That's a possibility! Sometimes there are things in the back of your mind that really affect how you think.

Sunday, May 18, 2008

Still in that Rut

This past week has been *super* hard for me. I'm not sure why or where this is coming from, nor am I sure if it's possible it might be because I've hit the midpoint of this transformation and I'm just getting bored or tired of it? Or is it the actual food? Or not being able to have my sweets or whatever else I want, like everyone else? It might be getting to my head more than usual lately. I DO NOT like at all how I've been feeling, almost like I'm stuck somewhere, for some reason with mixed feelings, and yet can't move either way. Strange. This is the first time throughout this transformation that I just feel lost. It's been a week that I've been dealing with feeling so much hungrier — sweets are getting to me — impatient, irritable, kind of everything at once. Usually, I'm strong with this stuff, mentally prepared, and have always gotten through it. Mind you, usually it would take only a day to pass, where this time it's been almost a week, on and off. Feels like a lifetime!

Today I've been extra irritable, not my usual self. I want to give in, but at the same time, I'm not sure to what? Sweets? Just to eating? I don't even know myself what I'm missing! I just know how I feel inside: down, low energy, somewhat depressed, and wanting to sleep off this crazy attitude. Yet, when I wake up, it's still there. I'm almost feeling as though I'm lost for some reason, as if I need someone to pick me up and get me excited again, to remind me why I'm doing all this and why it's important to finish it.

It's really strange to be in this spot right now. I always want answers why, why, why, and yet I cannot come up with the reason I'm feeling the way I have been. Is it boredom? Is it moving too

119

quickly for me? Are the sweets and foods I crave getting to me? Is it my diet that needs to be altered again? I really don't have an answer. I'm hoping for a better week next week. Meanwhile, I'll work my way through it.

Monday, May 19, 2008

Victoria Day Weigh-In

Another weigh-in day is here! I'm trying to keep positive that this week will be better than the last one regarding my emotional state.

This morning, when I weighed myself, to my surprise I had dropped a few more pounds. Honestly, after the week I've had, it's *something* to make me smile again.

This morning, the scale read 183 pounds, so I've dropped 4 pounds since last Monday. In total I've now written off 92 pounds since starting, which leaves me with 58 pounds to my final goal. I hope I can do this, friends! After the last week I had, believe me, I question my own strength.

I suppose I just have to remind myself to take it week by week like I've been doing. Not to allow myself to get overly anxious about the whole thing. That's the best way to tackle something like this. You can't allow yourself to look too far ahead. I know I need to give it all I've got each week, and *that* is what I need to focus on. Not the goal at the end!

That whole thought makes me happy. I've missed my sweets something terrible lately!

Monday, May 26, 2008

Another Milestone Is Fast Approaching

After weighing myself this morning, I was happy to see that I was able to lose another 3 pounds throughout the week that just passed. So I am standing at exactly 180 pounds on the dot. That leaves me now at a total weight loss of 95 pounds!

Last week was much better. Once again, I seem to be more balanced, where a week ago, I was all over the place emotionally, really questioning my strength regarding this whole thing.

It seems it was just the other day that I started this transformation project, not truly certain where I would end up, but carrying with me that one last ounce of hope that it would be different this time around. I trusted that my trainer would get me through this, once and for all. Well! Different it *has* been! I've never in my life been able to lose this amount of weight; I've never learned so much about the human body! My body has adapted very well, I think, to this whole new lifestyle. Compared to where my body was six and a half months ago, it's completely different!

From the beginning of this project, and even up until today, there were ideas in my mind that really stuck out, ideas that were different from those in the past, things like:

- For once in my life I was really able to look at where I actually stood, without covering up or trying to justify;
- I was able to take full blame, saying that "I" made (and kept making) some really bad

121

choices regarding my physical self; and
+ I was going to finally take action to fix it!

I believe these thoughts have made a huge difference in how I got through this so far.

And then I had to tackle the next phase, to mentally prepare myself to ACCEPT the fact that NOW I'll need to take what I did, and work really hard to do whatever it takes to turn it around and to restore and redo my body. This is something my body needs, and deserves!

Having these thoughts helped me prepare for what I was about to do. What I'm tackling right now has kept me on track ever since. I think this is really, really important! It's a huge thing to do (deciding to lose weight), but the proper frame of mind really does help get people though it.

When I'm finding it tough, or I'm having a bad day, or just sweating up a storm, I keep reminding myself that what I'm doing is the right thing to do, that I can never give up!

Thursday, May 29, 2008

Pushing Your Mind and Your Body Past the Limits . . .

I realize that not many people could stick to something like I've been doing. It's very strict. It tests the emotions. It's extremely tough at times, but it's made me strong. Seriously. This is the program my trainer goes on when he's training his body for a bodybuilding competition. I have no idea why he would want to do this every year. (In my view, once in your life is more than enough!) But a lot of people in this field do it. If anything, I've grown to appreciate the hard work bodybuilders go through. The women, too. I now have a taste of what it's like for them. By no means am I going to be a bodybuilder, but I can now understand the sweat and the hard work, and the mental toughness it entails. It's like pushing your mind and body *past* the limits of what you thought were the limits. There's the excitement of striving to get better and better. It's tough!

Friday, May 30, 2008

Run, Rosy, Run!
News!

I went to the gym with a friend, and when we started, we were warming up with our cardio . . . Well, to make a long story short: He started running. I chose to do the elliptical (as usual).

I said to him, "I can't do that yet. One day, but not yet."

But then something came over me and I thought, *I'm going to try this!* Once that thought got into my head, I just had to try it.

I stopped the elliptical, I got off, and I headed to the treadmill next to him. "If something happens to my knees, you're dead," I warned him.

I was just thinking while warming up with a walk, it's been so long I forget what it's like to run, but I just kept thinking good thoughts. (I guess I was trying to mentally prepare myself for what I was about to do.) *I should be able to do this by now. I can do this.* Then finally: "Here goes nothing!"

From a regular walk, I upped the speed to a brisk walk, then a little faster. (Felt weird knowing I was going to make myself try this.) Then once I was all warmed up? Off I went to the racetrack!

Man. It felt weird. I have a smile on my face just thinking about it. I kept going . . . and going . . .

It reminded me of the movie *Forest Gump*. Instead of saying "Run, Forest. Run," I was saying to myself "Run, Rosy. Run."

It was a rush, trying something new again! I could feel the intensity in my legs building as they began to burn, and I listened as my feet hit the mat so quickly over and over. All I could think was, *I'm running! I'm actually running!*

I wasn't sure if I should laugh or scream it out. I was just so amazed by the whole thing.

It was a great feeling. A moment to remember. In fact, I was so happy, I was close to continuing my run right off the end of that treadmill, right over to my friend — and anyone else who was in that gym — to give them all a big fat kiss!

I settled with telling my friend: "Look. You're the first to witness me doing this!" I believe he was happy too, and perhaps shocked as well. We continued our workout, and at the end, gave each other a big hug.

June 2008

Monday, June 2, 2008

Pulled Another 1-Pounder!

I cannot believe June has already arrived! But along with welcoming June, unfortunately, I also have to welcome one of those crappier weigh-in days, while facing the fact (and a reminder) that no matter how hard you work, sometimes the scale isn't always nice to you.

Scale showed 179 pounds this morning. One whole pound? *Man!* That's a bummer! Almost was hard to look at. *Damn,* I thought, and stepped off the scale, shrugging my shoulders. If anything, you'd think the run I did on Friday would have made me shed 10 pounds extra!

However . . . Throughout this transformation, I've learned that when my body does this — most of the time — it will make up for the lack of non-lost pounds the following week, and drop a few extra. So I hope this will be the case?

Sunday, June 8, 2008

Down in the Dumps

I don't think I'll be able to make the 100-pound mark for tomorrow's weigh-in. Perhaps Tuesday, but even that I'm not sure of. I've been looking at the scale throughout the week instead of waiting until Monday. It doesn't seem like it's going to be unless a miracle happens tonight.

I'm not upset as much as I'm disappointed. I really wanted this to be the big announcement, it might have to wait. Now that the temperature is rising lately, I'm afraid it's going to be more challenging to make myself get to that gym every day. The humidity makes me feel like I have no energy at all.

In the Meantime . . .

. . . to make myself feel better about how far I've come, I'm posting some pictures. I dug up some that were taken before I started the transformation project, and one was taken this past Saturday.

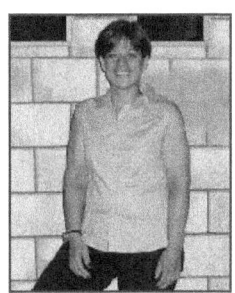

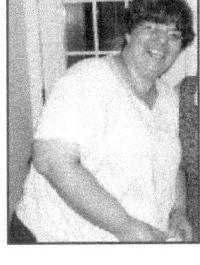

Since I'm that close — just a few pounds away — from the 100-pound total weight loss, I thought these would be more dramatic to help inspire others to change, or to keep them going if they've already started!

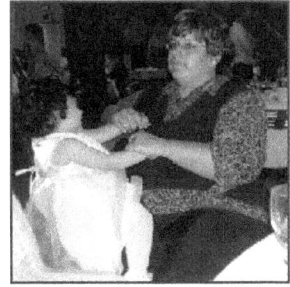

Monday, June 9, 2008

Weigh-In Day — Another Bad Week

It is very frustrating. I really believed that this week, I would have been able to reach that goal. To be 175 pounds. I've always set goals for myself, and have usually reached them within the time limit. This time around though, it hasn't been the case. I was totally off. I have no control over numbers. No matter how much I gave to get there, my body did not cooperate this time around.

I can't help but wonder why. I've been feeling heavier lately. Am I retaining water? Is this humidity holding that water in my body and not letting it out? Are my muscles weighing more? Is my body going to start giving me a hard time? Could it be that the stress I've been under lately is slowing down my metabolism? I really don't know. I will never know. There's been so much going on in my life these days, it's better I just leave this one alone and not add it to the list.

Why think about it? What's done is done. Not losing in numbers these past two weeks has really hit me, but I think it's only because I've been working extra hard at the gym trying to get to that certain milestone.

I guess we'll have to say my weight for today is 177 pounds. Another 1-pound loss since last week. How's that? There! I've written it down, I've accepted it. (It's hard to swallow.) So that brings me to a total weight loss of 98 pounds.

Wednesday, June 11, 2008

Seven-Month Pictures

Unfortunately I could not make the 100-pound weight loss goal. Still off by a few pounds. But that's okay. I could have lied, but since starting this, I've always been honest, and I'll continue to be honest right until the end.

So here are my recent pictures to compare with last month's.

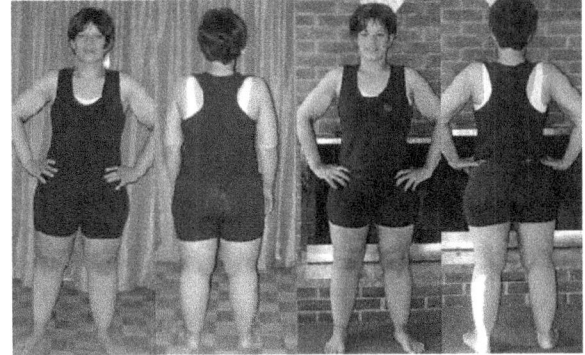

May   June

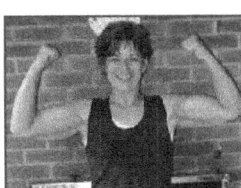

My legs look smaller this time! And my butt! Actually. Really. I think I shrunk everywhere a little.

Monday, June 16, 2008

Countdown to the Next Eat-All-The-Sweets-I-Want Day: Five Days

Weight today: 172 pounds.

I'm really proud of myself that I've stayed true to something for once in my life, dealing with the ups and downs of it all, while staying firm, focused, and determined, without losing sight of one thing: that I WILL get to my goal!

Probably for the first time ever, I've taken control of a situation without letting life's stresses take it away from me for one reason or another. What's the saying? "Come hell or high water"? In my case, that's what I feel like. Life could have shot anything at me, but this time around, I was coming out a winner in this fight against obesity!

Everything in your life becomes different when you lose a lot of weight. Before, my life was more about being happy with whatever I could get (settling) instead of having the choice of what "I" wanted.

This concerns several aspects of my life. I'm not talking only about clothes, et cetera. It goes way beyond that. When I look back over the years, starting in high school, I feel like that's what my life was based on: "Be happy and thankful with whatever you can get." Sad, but true.

Now I have choices — although I'll have to admit, it's kind of scary at times. And I can find myself feeling guilty because now I spend time on "me" sometimes, rather than on family.

In the past, I was always at home, always around, wearing my jogging pants and my T-shirt, making great tasty suppers, baking delicious sweets, just going through my daily life doing things for others. Assuming I was happy. I would never buy anything for me, or very rarely if I did, and usually, it would just be the necessities.

But now that's all changed.

I go out with friends. Sometimes, you can find me in the makeup aisle at the drug store. I watch for specials on clothes. (I have patience now to try new things on.) I shop for shoes. That was never me before, but I guess when you start feeling good about yourself, you start caring about the different aspects of you, how you're dressing, how you present yourself.

Anyway, I'm just trying to stay grounded while dealing with all these things on a completely different scale. My life was routine, I always knew what was going to happen. Now? It's so different, I really never know!

When you've been a certain way for most of your life and all of a sudden, within seven months, your life changes completely, it's shocking. What happened to my other life? It's like waking up one morning and things have changed. I'm sure people can understand why I find it scary. Emotionally, you're dealing with trying to figure it all out at the same time as you're trying to put it all into place.

Friday, June 20, 2008

One Hour to Go until My Cheat Day

(... a little secret, though: I got a head start on it. My trainer won't be impressed.)

I admit to going to Dairy Queen with my sister and her kids earlier tonight! I ordered ice cream. It's on my list of favourites. Tomorrow is my Cheat Day, but I just couldn't resist starting early.

What did I have? I decided to have one of those advertised new features, the Fudge Brownie Temptation Waffle Bowl Sundae. And when I was asked by the young girl if I wanted the waffle dipped in chocolate, I responded with a huge smile, "OF COURSE!" And boy, was it chocolaty!

At first — for the first two minutes — I really did enjoy it. All that fudge and whipped cream and brownie chunks. It was a taste that brought back many good feelings. However, as I kept eating it, I started feeling not so good, something that was also familiar to me from my past eating habits, the feeling that you just ate WAY too much of something, and you just feel sick. What? Sick? That WASN'T part of the plan. Talk about putting a damper on my plans to go nuts at DQ!

I couldn't finish it!

At least it was a thrill for me to have been able to order it, something others might take for granted. Rarely have I had even *that* opportunity in the last seven months.

And since it was SO chocolaty, I wasn't sure I'd want any other sweets tomorrow. But tomorrow is a whole new day, and time will tell. I have my liquorice stashed in a cupboard downstairs so I can rip it open tomorrow morning, if I choose to.

Even though I cheated early, I feel I deserved every bite! I've worked so hard, mentally and physically all these months, what's a few hours? Not much when you look at the big picture. Besides, I was able to wait months for this moment to arrive, so you know what? *Who cares!*

Monday, June 23, 2008

The Monday after the Weekend Cheat

Weight today: 171 pounds.

Looks like the downfall of my Cheat Day is that I gained 2 pounds from it. Friday I took note for fun, that I weighed 169 pounds, so it did set me back a little. But no problem, today is only Monday. I'm sure I'll be back down by next weigh-in. Let's hope the world doesn't start heating up again and I start retaining water . . . Can't be doing that to me now!

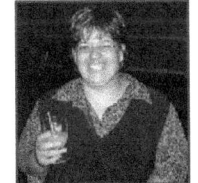

I'm posting a couple of photos from the night of my party.

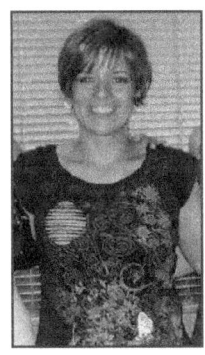

Oh, I just *had* to add in the old picture, too.

The old picture was taken at the high school reunion I organized back in September, so two months before starting. I remember thinking I looked

133

really good that night. But I had to post it, because to me (I don't know about you) it DOES NOT look like the same person. I thought it would be fun to compare.

The one with the cake is my favourite because it doesn't need any words. The expression on my face truly shows the excitement and joy one feels when you work hard trying to get to a goal, and you reach an important milestone on the way!

Makes me tear up looking at the picture with the cake. It's how I've really been feeling lately.

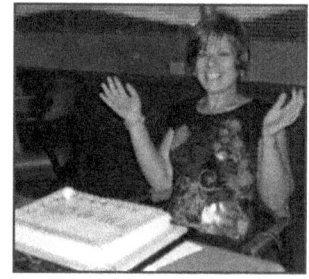

(The cake was reflecting the numbers the scale read on the Friday: 169 pounds = 105 pounds lost.)

Friday, June 27, 2008

I'm Front Page News!

You're probably wondering what it's like when I hit the front page. Is it exciting for her? What goes through her mind?

First of all, it was a surprise for me as well! The *Ottawa Sun* doesn't tell me when I'm on the front page. I was aware that another article was going to be inside the *Sun*, but that's all I knew. They seem to leave that out for some reason. Not sure if it's on purpose to make it a special surprise for me or what, but, today's edition was a little more special to me, regardless.

I just looked at it thinking, *gawd,* that's really me!
I'm actually on the front page again! Sometimes it
just makes you feel like you're dreaming it or
something, but yet, it's really you in that picture.
And for a moment, a "proudness" came over me
as I was reading it. (It was a really nice feeling,
actually.) I just cannot believe that I'm really
almost there! At the end! And that this is really
happening in my life for the very first time. That
I've come face to face with this problem I had for
so long, and I'm defeating it!

I never would have thought, only months ago,
that my life was about to take such a different
direction and change so drastically. However, the
greatest part of this whole project is the hope that
I'm inspiring others by going public about it,
giving them a chance to see for themselves that it
really can be done by a normal person.

I've been able to take steps toward changing my
life to make it a better one, health-wise, at least,
while perhaps helping someone else in the
process. That makes me the best damn
housekeeper around.

Lately I've been feeling like my story has all of a
sudden been touching a lot of people.

Perhaps it's because I've been so honest during
this whole project, refusing to hide anything.
Maybe people appreciate my honesty, allowing
them to get inside my mind throughout it, rather
than just showing Before and After shots.

I'll always care about and respect people who are
overweight/obese because I know how hard it
can be to live that life! Once you've lived it, you

can never forget. It gives you the ability to see past
the physical side that other people see. People
can't hide being overweight, but whether they
choose to admit it or not, it can be a hard and even
a sad life at times.

I *know* being obese can be both a hard and a sad
life at times, because I lived that life for so long.
When we make the choice to change, and just do
it, you finally get a taste of what it's like to be on
the other side, as in my case. It's almost surreal
because it's so different, but you finally feel free.
That's the only way to describe it, feeling free, like
nothing can hold you back anymore!

What's also sad is, even though I've lost a lot of
weight, why was I not as special in people's eyes
before? You know what I mean. It was still me.
Same person. Life is kind of sad that way, isn't it?
It's real though. And true.

We are all special you know, no matter what
shape we are in. It's all about making a choice and
working toward a goal. Make that choice only
when you are really ready to make a change in
your life, no matter what that might be. But never
give up until you reach your goal!

Want to hear something funny? When we first
broke the news about this project, most people
just thought, nice story, but they won't do it, she'll
fail. And so the question was: Will she be able to
do it or not? Maybe some people were just waiting
for me to fail, but I think I've changed their
thoughts on that.

And yet, now that we are showing people we *are*
doing it and that it will be done, the question

people are now asking is: Will she be able to maintain it?

You all should know me by now! So far, everything I promised you I would do, I have done, so I can tell you right now that I WILL maintain it. I've worked *way* too hard to get here to not do that.

The best thing about this project though, is that it shows you what we all have — no matter where we are right now — and that's the inner strength to change or to defeat anything that has held us back. It's a wonderful power that we are ALL given! Mentally, we're very strong; it's what we do with that strength that's key. So among other things, this project proves that point, to each of us.

Monday, June 30, 2008

110 Pounds Down. 40 to Go!

Here are my numbers for today . . .

Today's weight: 165 pounds; last Monday's weight: 171 pounds; total weight loss to date: 110 pounds!

I'm really happy about numbers this morning. I'm at the exact point where I have 40 pounds left to lose. It's nice, especially since we are on a timed mission!

So far, we're right on target, I think. Things are going fairly smoothly. I have four months and a bit left in the transformation, so if I can lose 10 pounds a month from here on in, we'll be okay. That's just around the corner!

How exciting is that! I mean, I might be able to show the world that it's possible for people to lose 150 pounds in just one year, by eating well and exercising. Incredible.

I can still remember last November like it was yesterday. It was cold, there was a lot of snow. While the rest of the world slept all snuggled and warm, I was out there at 6:00 in the morning, cursing, as I brushed off and scraped my car, getting it ready to get to my gym . . . And now? I'm almost at the finish line! Wow! WOW!

I just cannot believe it. Where did the time go?

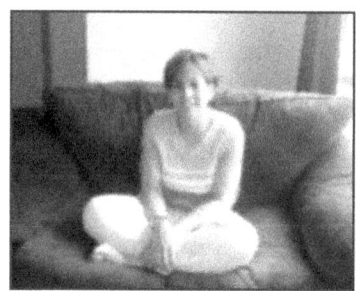

July 2008

Wednesday, July 2, 2008

Stop Letting Your Weight Ruin Your Life

The other night, I was talking to Jay (a friend from the gym, who has also lost over 100 pounds alone). He is just so great to talk with. We can really relate on this topic of losing weight, and where we stand right now, and what life is like compared to before.

Last night, while having our regular chat on the computer, I told him something I feel strongly about: When I was so overweight in the past, being big like that robbed me. It took from my life what should have been mine! That is the saddest part. I missed out on so much over the years, and as the days keep passing and I'm starting to challenge myself at new things, I see it.

Take a moment to think about that because it's SO true, perhaps more than we want to believe, or admit to ourselves.

Yesterday I went out with the kids, and I did something I never thought I would do. I went on this climbing ride. It was so much fun. The people I went with didn't want to go on the ride, so the girls said to me: "You're the smallest. You go." So I went. It was an amazing feeling. To go. To get up there. To not be shy. To just enjoy it! To fit. To laugh. It's so amazing when you start enjoying things you never tried before (because your weight stood in the way).

Another topic Jay and I discussed was that while I was there, I noticed so many people who were eating really bad, bad foods, almost overloading on them, not realizing what they were doing to

140

themselves, what they were putting into their mouths. I did not judge them, I really am not like that, but most of these people were pretty large, and I thought if only they knew what they were doing to themselves — or better yet, if only they could understand that by continuing to do this, they were deciding to take a lot away from their lives. If only they cared enough to take control.

It was almost sad to me now that I've pretty much defeated this problem myself. You start seeing things in a new light. I used to be the woman who was sitting there eating a huge hot dog and a large poutine as if there wasn't a problem, not realizing that I was living my life to eat — or living my life to *die* if I kept going at that rate.

Anyway, I had to write about that. If you have a weight problem, think about what I said. Lose weight first of all for yourself and your health. Get angry about robbing yourself of enjoying things because you're too heavy, or if you feel you might not fit into something, or if you automatically avoid situations altogether. You miss out on so much. No, it isn't fair, but it's never too late! You deserve this life, just like I do! We all deserve to live a rich, happy, healthy life. I know, for myself, the "fat" life I once lived — comparing it to now — well, I tell you, emotionally I don't have that weight holding me down anymore. Believe me that makes a *huge* difference. It changes your life completely, how you view things, the new things you can do. You challenge yourself. Your smile is much more genuine because you're actually happy inside. I can write a list of the differences between the fat life and a healthy life.

I hope this topic will help motivate you, and give you more reasons to change. I know for myself in the past, even when I dated a boyfriend and he was a jerk and I wanted to get over him, I would make myself get MAD. I would think about what a real jerk he was and start putting him down a lot, picking out all his flaws . . . just basically begin to hate him, and that helped.

So begin by getting mad. That's a start. Use that anger to change. Remember: You *deserve this*! Just like everyone else. And if you take some time to start changing how you eat, making healthier choices, and letting exercise become part of your life, you'll find yourself on the right path to your own life, the one YOU have chosen to take back!

Monday, July 7, 2008

Weigh-In

My weight this morning was 166 pounds. So the scale says I went up a pound since last Monday.

Doesn't bother me whatsoever though, because I know I haven't given in to anything. Still sailing along. Keep in mind, though, that last week I did lose a lot as far as numbers went, so it could just be balancing out. Since starting this transformation project, that is one thing I've noticed. On the whole, usually you don't see two great weeks of dropping. So it's all good.

I've been really, really happy lately. Almost like I've been on this natural high. Not sure why, not sure what's causing it, but I'm loving every minute. I find I've just been feeling different. Kind of weird.

This Friday is picture day! I can't believe another month has come and gone already. Wow. I can't wait to see these ones and what they show.

Wednesday, July 9, 2008

Here We Go with the Humidity . . .

Lately it's been really humid. With the humidity, I tend to have a hard time finding my energy. I walk around feeling heavy, as if my legs are two sacs of cement. I hate that.

Also, my appetite has gone up in the last few days, and when that happens, so do my cravings for sweets. Last night I was thinking of chocolate cake, ice cream . . . *Mmm.* I think it's to do with the weather because I don't tend to get cravings as much anymore, as long as I'm feeling satisfied (enough food).

I will just have to deal with it. I'm almost at the end of this now. I couldn't possibly allow myself to get weak at this point in the game, that would be plain stupid. I'm so excited anticipating the end when the best is yet to come. Whatever will I look like? This transformation has been so amazing so far, I can't even imagine what I'll look like in November when I can proudly say that I made it, I did it, for the very first time in my life I succeeded! After all the hard work I will have put myself through for twelve months, I will finally get to reap the reward of a brand new life!

My trainer is going to have some surprises in store for me after August, when we are down to the last three months. I'm kind of scared about what that might be. I have a feeling he's going to work me even harder, perhaps the hardest ever, and put me on certain diets that I might find extra tough. It's scary, but exciting at the same time.

Friday, July 11, 2008

Seven- and Eight-Month Pictures to Compare

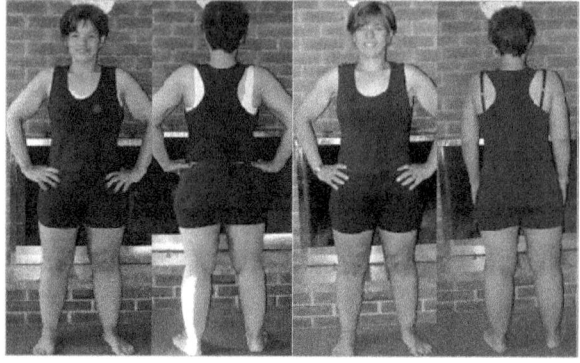

June   July

Well I have to say, I don't see much of a difference this morning. I don't know why that is, but here they are, just the same.

I'm mad right now. I look at these photos and I think *garbage*. To me they are the worst photos taken yet. After working out really hard for five days out of each week, for four weeks, that's *all* the change I get? That's if you want to even call it a change because I know I sure don't.

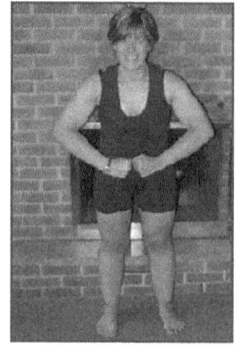

Boy, do I feel ripped off right now. And frustrated. Like I said, worst photos ever! So I'm not going to be having a good day today!

144

Sunday, July 13, 2008

Ready to Tackle a Brand New Week
. . . and the Start of a Kick-Butt Month

Weight, 163 pounds. I'm hoping to be in the 150s in the next few weeks.

I had time to think about the last post where I mentioned that I was a little disappointed in my photos (okay, *really* disappointed). At first I could not see much change, but after looking at them a few times, I suppose there were some changes.

It surprised me. Until now, every time I posted my monthly photos, there was a significant change. Thinking about it now, with my head clear, with only 38 pounds left to lose, I know that's good. Not much more will happen now . . . only more toning, I guess, and muscle building.

That being said, I'm now getting myself ready to tackle a whole new month starting tomorrow, before my last pictures to compare are posted on August 11. Once again, I plan to give it all I can until then, and hope for the best.

I still can't believe how close I am now to reaching the end. I'm really shocked. I've mentally been able to stay focused and strong enough to keep this thing going. I have not once thought about quitting. Standing here today, I think I've grown as a person by doing this project.

Looking at my current photos, I find it hard to believe it's me, Rosy, that I'm seeing. Who is this new person and where did she come from? I was big for most of my life, and with all the extra weight gone, I'm left looking at a whole new person, almost a stranger I'm just starting to get to know: a stronger, focused, Ready-To-Tackle-Anything-That-Comes-Her-Way type of woman.

I sometimes wonder how my life will be from here on in, now that I'm so completely different from a physical and mental standpoint. Unlike in the past, I don't have anything standing in my way. Now, I can reach for the stars if I want to.

It's funny, but when I look at any one of my old pictures, I want to hug that person before I say (with great relief) that final goodbye. That person went through a lot emotionally from being overweight all those years. I'll still always have the sad memories of that life. No amount of weight loss can erase those. But, at the same time I'm proud of myself that, somehow, I made it through. I never would have thought there would come a day when I'd be sitting here, writing for people around the world. Something that started off as a mere idea has gone far! I made a promise to myself, and I kept it. Even if I were to stay exactly here, at this point, where I am right now, I'd still be very happy.

What the next months bring in the way of training will be an extra for you, really. At the same time, it will give me a chance to challenge my own body on another level once again. It might be brutal, it might be tough, it might even test my emotional capacity to the extreme, but with the greatest trainer and friend by my side, I'm ready for it! So together let's do it and finish this thing!

(I might change my attitude when he gives me my new training and diet later in August, but you know me, I'm a fighter. Right to the end.)

Monday, July 21, 2008

Weigh-In

Today's weight 160 pounds. Down 3 since last week.

Monday, July 28, 2008

Weigh-In

Today's weight 157 pounds!

Total of 118 pounds lost to date

I have 32 pounds to go!

As you can see from the numbers, I've dropped another 3 pounds since last Monday. I'm pretty happy with that number. I'm including a picture taken on Saturday night when I went out with "the girls." I really like including pictures like this from time to time because I think it reminds everyone that I'm a real live person. I don't have to always submit just my monthly pictures with the same clothes on, or in which I'm flexing my muscles for all to see how they are developing. I'm normal, too!

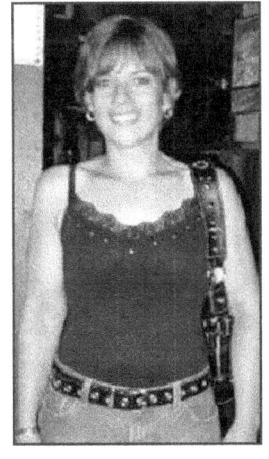

I do go out like you and other people do, and I do get ready to go out as well. It's easier now that I'm beginning to fit into different sorts of clothes,

clothes that at one time I never thought I would *ever* look good in! But that has changed. I'm starting to get gutsy in a lot of ways.

I'm starting to get more comfortable wearing tight-fitting clothes. When I first put on this outfit on Saturday, I was paranoid! I was questioning if my butt looked big, or if my stomach showed, but as the day went on, it got better.

Now that I have control of my eating, it's easy. After a while, you just know what you should be eating or not eating. That's the greatest. It really does become the norm for you, and you'll not look at it as a hassle anymore.

Food can actually make us crazy. I remember that all too well. When we're hungry, it takes us over. We become different people when we're weak, jumping at the first thing we see, and finding ourselves *over*eating as well, not to mention eating garbage: stuff soaked in oil, high in sodium, made with strange ingredients. I don't know about you, but I never understood exactly what half of those things listed were. That's scary.

The first part of healing and making changes is to ADMIT where you stand. That means, getting the guts and the courage to tell people around you how much you weigh. That was really, really hard for me in the beginning. It was a secret I had carried around with me for years. But when the day came to make a change, the first thing I did was tell people my weight. For me to be able to say it, and hear it, and accept it, was very important. When I did that, I think I began to heal.

Then, I immediately stopped — and I mean COMPLETELY stopped — eating those bad foods. If it wasn't naturally grown, or actually unprocessed chicken meat and turkey meat, it was never going to enter this body again! I stopped drinking juices and began eating real fresh fruit, making great salads; my morning cereals were organic, and natural, without the sugars and other things many cereals have. I watched my portions, I started to prepare my foods in advance so I'd always have my healthy food on hand in the fridge. That's it. I made a choice to change.

That's what it's all about. Make a choice to change, and STICK TO IT, no matter what. Even when you feel weak, you have to keep it going!

For the first few weeks, until you get those addictive foods out of your system, it's tough. You need a friend or someone to talk to during this time. You need to have them commit to helping you when you get weak. It will be their job to get you out of that state. They can be that person who reminds you of *why* you chose to change, and that NO, you don't *need* that bad food; that it's not a big deal to not have it even though at that point in time you may feel like you need it so badly. Make sure the person you choose is ready to take on that role. It must be someone strong. It would make no sense at all to have someone as weak as you are, who will say "Oh well, one day won't hurt." IT DOES HURT. In the beginning! One day will turn into two, then three, and so on. Avoiding those foods completely — it might be the hardest thing to do at first — in itself will make you strong later! You're helping your body to get rid of the stuff that made you fat to begin with. Next, you'll start to nourish your body the way you should have been doing. IT'S NEVER TOO LATE FOR THAT.

And get to that gym! Get physical. Even today, I still have times when I just don't feel like going. But having become mentally stronger, I know I have no choice but to go, so I get myself there even if I have to drag my feet along the way. Once you're there, it's not that bad. It's one hour out of your day. The faster you're in, the faster you're out. Makes it harder when you think of it as a hassle. Try to think of it as something you have to do. End of story. No ifs, ands, or buts about it.

Now get going and start to change! I need to make my breakfast, and lunch for that matter, oh, and do some laundry, too, and get my daughter up, get her to the daycare, and get to the gym . . . and the list goes on, and on.

August 2008

Sunday, August 3, 2008

In the Dieting World, It's All about Control

CONTROL is something I've learned through this project. It's something we ALL can learn. It becomes the norm after a while, it becomes part of you. You just know, eventually, that you *do* have to make time to prepare your own stuff! You also know that you do not need to eat leftovers like you once did. Weird, eh? It's great to be able to do that. It makes your life so much easier, and you feel good inside. It makes you *mentally* strong!

It's always going to be hard at first, but with time, things get easier. Who wouldn't *love* to be in control of what they're eating, and how they see food. I think everyone would like that, and it's something we all *can* do. Give it a chance. By doing it, and by practising control, you'll be starting a whole new life for yourself!

Sunday, August 10, 2008

Nine-Month Anniversary Pictures

Transformation Project: It's Crunch Time

Well these are my newest pictures taken tonight. That's right. My nine-month pictures. I just decided that instead of posting all the pictures, why not just the originals with the newest. Makes it more dramatic now, doesn't it? It's almost like it's not even the same person when looking at it.

Now you have to ask yourself, What have I been doing for the past nine months? Do you guys see now, just how fast nine months go by? And what a dramatic change someone can make within that time?

If I had chosen to do nothing, I'd probably still look like those November 2007 pictures. Imagine! How sad if I'd decided to stay there. I mean look at me. Do I look happy? I don't think so.

I decided to take action! I've included extra pictures so you can see I'm in the best shape I've ever been in. I can't even believe it myself.

The choice is in your hands. You can change like this, too, if you want to. It depends on how badly you want it. Will you let the foods take over and win? Or will you put a stop to it today and start a new life? A healthier and happier life? Do it! You CAN do it!

This was done NATURALLY with no pills, no surgery, nothing except hard work and

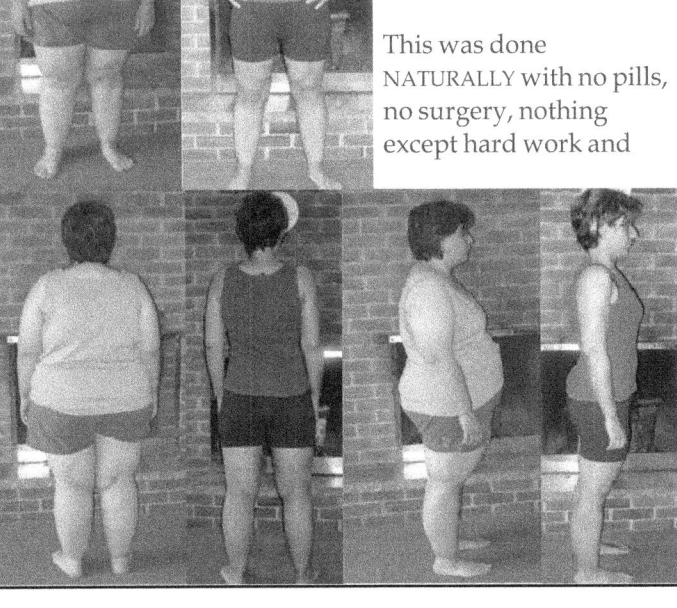

discipline, eating better foods, and exercising five times a week. Again, in only nine months!

My three-month intense training starts in the morning. I'll be off to the gym earlier tomorrow trying to get through this brand new routine! Well, I hope you enjoy these pictures because they'll be the *last* ones you'll see until the end in November. I need to leave you guys wondering, I can't give it all away.

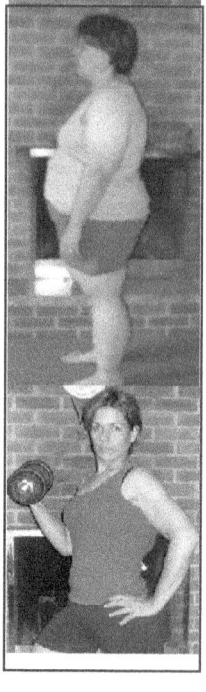

Don't Allow Yourself to Waste Time Caring What Others Think!

These last few days have really tested my mental strength and my control over food. There have been a few

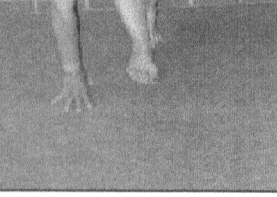

issues that I've had to deal with throughout this past month, on different levels, and during these last few days, I've had this hunger for something other than my own food!

It's strange how our bodies react like that. When you're dealing with issues that are taking an emotional toll on you, you tend to all of a sudden feel hungry, and want to eat.

I've been able to control it however, because I now know, after doing this for nine months, that you have to just keep going. Maintain control, no matter what! You can not allow people, nor stressful situations, to bring you down, nor let anything cloud your mind about what you set out to do. You cannot allow THAT to be your excuse to deny yourself of what you REALLY want. YOU are too important. No matter what, you have to keep your head up high while you continue the fight.

It's extremely easy, even for me, to reach for something bad. For example, I have to shop for groceries today. I already know I'll be looking at junk food, everywhere, screaming "BUY ME!"

It doesn't help that I'm down to the last bit of weight. At times, the only thing stopping me from buying and eating junk food is the "time" issue of all this. Where I stand weight-wise now, if I wanted to, I *could* have something bad one day. It wouldn't hurt me. But I know I only have a certain amount of weeks left (fifteen) to get to the goal we set out to attain — which was to prove to every one every where that you CAN lose 150 pounds in just one year, naturally. I can't afford to take a chance on the outcome. Doesn't that suck?)

But hey! Fifteen weeks. That's not much! That puts a smile on my face, that's for sure — and provides a sense of relief. I feel I've already defeated this obesity problem, because I've already begun to enjoy my new life.

I know with my birthday coming up in about five weeks, September 11, I plan to have a HUGE piece of cake, no matter what anyone says! It will be the start of a whole new year (new life!) for me! A completely different one from the ones I was used to in the past. And you can bet that when I blow out those candles, I'll be saying GOODBYE to the old life I led for so many years, and I'll be wishing for many new wonderful things to come my way. I wonder if I can have thirty-four wishes? One for each year to make up for the years I never wished for anything. (Okay. So maybe I'm asking too much from the birthday angel.)

Monday, August 11, 2008

Weigh-In & Summary of One Routine

This morning's reading on the scale was 153 pounds. I'm looking forward to getting down to the 140s *soon*! I can't wait!

To be exact, there are only *thirteen weeks and two days* before we get to November 11. I can't believe it! Where did the time go? By the time August is over, we'll be counting this baby down BIG TIME!

I'm excited and nervous at the same time as I wonder if I'll be able to reach my goal of being 125 pounds in twelve months. A number I've never, *ever* been since childhood. All I can say is: I'll give it all I've got to get there! I'll have to lose 28 pounds during these next thirteen weeks.

Friday, August 15, 2008

iReport for CNN

News! The producer of CNN said they liked my story so much they want my story and pictures as one of their listed features. I don't believe many get picked for that, so I was really flattered when I was asked. I'm one out of only seven! And you know what's really cool? I'm the only one from *Canada*! How cool is that? *Yes! We did it!*

Sunday, August 17, 2008

Weight Today: 151 Pounds!

<u>Only Twelve Weeks Left . . .</u>
Weight today: 151 pounds.

Total pounds lost to date: 124!

Total pounds left to lose: 26!

With twelve weeks left in this transformation project, I do not have time to be weak or get caught up in frustration. I have to bite the bullet and go at it full force, even though it's taking everything I have.

I suppose this is where all the months of mentally challenging myself will come into play. It really is a mental game. If you have the proper mind set, you can get past anything!

Even though I would say now: "Yes. I'm a much stronger person both physically and mentally than I once was," the real question is, how *much* stronger am I? How *much* can I take without breaking?

With all the hours I've already endured at the gym, along with the diets, how can I possibly find the mental strength to work even harder? To actually see myself through this final phase, and to actually be able to wrap this whole thing up?

Rob had warned me that the final three months of this project would be the toughest ever. That they would really test my limits. To be honest, I'm starting to feel it, and we've only just begun!

At the gym now, I have to mentally shut out every thing and every one around me so I can aim my energy and my focus onto each and every workout exercise. I must make myself step it up a notch, enter into a whole different level of training.

Monday, August 25, 2008

Just When You Think You're Alone . . .

Sometimes, even though, at the time, you think you're alone, really, you're not. And in those times of need, all of a sudden everyone comes out to lend a hand, or to say nice things, and it means so much.

This morning started off tough. Emotionally. I was upset. It took everything to get myself to my routine. But surprisingly, once I was there, it wasn't as bad as I thought it would be. Perhaps because it helped take my mind off the frustration I was feeling.

I told my trainer (in person this time, which was really nice, something I think I needed): "If I were to stay where I am right now, I would honestly be happy. I've come so far and, right now, I know I would be looked upon as being happy and healthy." But I guess sometimes you make personal goals for yourself, and this 125-pound thing is just my personal goal. It's something I really believe deep down that I (we) can achieve and get to, and that's what I'm anxiously awaiting.

Now that we're getting closer to the end, I'll be getting frustrated and nervous. Can we do it? Will we do it?

Rob said that this goal I've had since the beginning is probably what has kept me going until now, just visualizing that 125-pound mark on the scale that I believed (and still believe) I'd see one day. I never lost sight of that, never stopped visualizing it. It was, and is, something I've never had a chance to experience in my life! To be seen as "normal." No more terms like "obese" — or worse, "morbidly obese" (which is what I was health-wise).

I hate those two words: "morbid" and "obese." I cannot stand saying those words, or hearing them, or even writing them! They are so degrading! I wish they could be erased from the dictionary.

Now I don't want people to take things the wrong way when I get upset, and maybe think to themselves: *Oh look at her. She's getting all obsessed now. She should be happy where she's at. Why is she complaining?* It's not at all about that. I just want to make it. That's all. For myself. So I can say: "Look. I did it!" I want this so badly now, more than ever, and I've had it in the back of my mind this whole time, since last November, to get to that goal in twelve months . . . and I just want to make it!

This is the last final goal that I'm working toward. Remember in the beginning when I used to always say "Make smaller goals at first and they'll help time pass, et cetera, and before you know it, you'll be there"? Well, I've passed all those smaller goals. Now, I just want to get to the biggest, final one.

In the meantime, big thanks go to my trainer, my family, my friends, and all of you. If I didn't have this kind of support, I'm not sure I could have stuck with it this long.

I still believe what makes a big difference in the outcome in weight loss is where you're at mentally. If people can get the mental part down, it's a lot easier. That mental strength is what will get you past what I went through this morning.

And this morning was a *really* bad one. Probably the worst one yet. During the months that have passed, I think Rob has really prepared me, by being so tough, and strict, and I think I'm strong enough to get through anything now. No matter how I felt today, I not once thought about eating bad foods. That's impressive, and I think it says a lot about how tough I really am now, compared with before.

I'm feeling a lot better tonight! My meeting with Rob went really well. We'll be changing the diet somewhat, and it's just great to get reassured once again. I think that's all I really needed.

It was so nice to get online and see the posts coming up in my email from all of you. So great to hear from friends who really care, even when I'm not at my happiest.

Saturday, August 30, 2008

Some Days You Just Need to Get Back to Your Roots

I promised I'd always be honest with you, so I have to tell you that on Thursday night, once everything was calm in the house, and the kids were in bed, I sent my husband out to get me a

Peanut Buster Parfait from our friends over at Dairy Queen. That's right. I sure did! Not a small one either to split the calories, I ordered the regular one! And, to top it off, once I ate that up, I decided to get into the Doritos nacho chips too! Yup! So here I am to confess my sins.

While eating them, I thought (smiling to myself) *Oh my. If only Rob could see me now . . . If only the world could see me now, making a personal choice like this without anyone okaying it, and enjoying all this vanilla ice cream with what seemed like mounds of hot chocolate fudge* (it's almost like they knew it was for me because there was even more than usual) *and peanuts . . .* I tell ya it was so YUMMY!

That has always been my favourite Dairy Queen treat. I've been getting the Peanut Buster Parfait for years, probably since I was thirteen years old. The funny thing is, I don't really know why I wanted it.

Its not that I got weak, it's not that I was having a bad day, I just had an urge for it. Perhaps it's because since my kids have been back from out of town, life has been so on-the-go for me, so chaotic. If I were to tell you how my days actually go, I wouldn't know where to start. The truth is, I haven't had much, if any, time just for *me* lately. I'm not even sure how I do it sometimes, balancing everything that goes on all at once.

Thursday night, I just wanted some time for me. To enjoy something that *I* really like. I didn't feel bad about it either. I've been working out so hard lately (on top of everything else), that I thought I deserved it, no matter what the scale read.

Once you get something like that out of your system, automatically you think *Okay. How am I going to burn this off now?* Yes it was good. But yet . . . oh so *bad*!

Sunday, August 31, 2008

So Now I'm Broke . . .

What a hectic Sunday! I cannot believe what a rush today was. With the holiday tomorrow, I wanted to get any last-minute school shopping out of the way, so I had to run to quite a few stores picking up things that were on special, and any last-minute items they needed. During the drive home, the kids and I were pooped, and I was thinking about how broke I was, just like many other mothers out there when it's back-to-school time. But the kids were happy.

September 2008

Monday, September 1, 2008

Welcome to the World of the 140s. Finally!

Today's weight: 149 pounds.

Total weight loss to date: 126 pounds.

Weight left to lose: 24 pounds to go!

Phew! Okay!

So this morning the scale read 149 pounds. Finally! *Man!* I waited a long time to see that needle drop below the 150 zone! What a relief.

Hopefully, my trainer and I finally cracked that code and we are back to losing some weight again, and that from this point on, the numbers will continue to drop more smoothly. That was a long wait this time around! Longest EVER I think, since starting this whole thing. The numbers would not budge, no matter what.

Ten weeks. Ten weeks. Ten weeks. Ten weeks. I can't believe it when I write that! It puts a big huge smile on this girl's face.

Something Funny
The other night I went to bingo with my mom. It was ages since I did that. My mom enjoys my company, so I decided to go with her this time.

Although I didn't have many chances at winning that night, while we were there, my mom (being the mom she is, like many other moms) had to point out to a few of her bingo friends that the daughter who's been in the *Ottawa Sun* — "the one who's lost all the weight?" — was there with her that night. Believe it or not, there were people there who had been following my story! So I got a lot of smiles and hellos. *(Oh, Mother!* I thought to myself. *Talk about embarrassing!)*

Anyway, when we were outside on a break, there was this older Spanish lady my mom talks to and who takes the bus with her sometimes. She doesn't speak that well in English, usually combines English and Spanish. But with me being Italian, I'm used to combined things. Italians do it all the time.

So my mom says to this woman: "Guess how old my daughter is."

My mom whispers to me: "Let's see how old she thinks you are." She's smiling, thinking that the lady will definitely say a younger age, right? No doubt about that one!

What does the lady respond with? "Forty-three."

"Huh?" You should have seen the reaction on my mom's face. "Forty-three? No, no, no, no."

I just smiled and chuckled. I've never been told I look forty-three. These days, people think I'm in my twenties.

Thursday, September 4, 2008

Things Are Going Well

Mentally, I've been feeling great, lots of energy while I visualize and focus on the end. I'm trying to pretend I'm already in November.

I had three people come up to me this week to tell me how I've changed, and I didn't even know them well! I suppose you never know who's watching you. You think no one is, but then all of a sudden, a stranger will approach you and tell you (sincerely, too) how great you look, and how far you've come. That really IS something nice to hear from time to time.

Monday, September 8, 2008

Another Busy Week Ahead

Today's weight: 144 pounds.

Weight left to lose: 19 pounds.

Time left: nine weeks and one day. (Countdown time! *Tick tock, tick tock.*)

As you can see, it's going a little more smoothly lately with the weight. It seems to be dropping since the last plateau. (Thank goodness.)

So we are on track!

I woke up this morning thinking *Oh my. It's going to be a busy week for me. And where do I start?*

Well. I guess I'll start by getting up and just getting through it. Not much else you *can* do.

Life has been so on the go for me lately. Monday to Friday, it's like doing a relay race all day long trying to fit everything into one day. You can bet on it that I look forward to MY weekends, to slow myself down, to relax, to give my mind a break. But as I said in one of my past entries, we *are* at the end now. Only a few weeks left. Before you know it, those weeks, too, will all have come and gone. I can just see myself looking back, wondering where the time went, when I've completed my mission.

My birthday is coming up on Thursday! I see it as a special one. That's why I'm mentioning it a lot. It's the start of a new year for me, a brand new life for the years that follow! (So, I guess I should have at least one piece of cake . . .) I really don't want to ruin where I am today as far as weight goes, but as long as that's all I have, I should be okay.

Thursday, September 11, 2008

A Little Overboard

Okay. So I went just a little overboard for my birthday night.

I'm sure I'll disappoint some of you with the details of my birthday night. I know there were a few of you who said "Don't eat the cake," but guess what? You know me. I did. *And* some! Sometimes I can be stubborn.

First of all, I had a meeting with my trainer tonight. We went to a really nice Italian bakery in the Little Italy district here in Ottawa, to discuss an upcoming project we are now working on. Can't tell you about it just yet, but I think it will make some of you REALLY, REALLY happy down the road.

Anyway, I kind of failed to tell him that I started to eat a little earlier, prior to meeting him. So, Rob, if you're reading this, I'm sorry.

I started mid-afternoon. When he asked me after our "meeting" if I could control myself if we chose to eat one piece of cake and a nice *biscotti*, I said "Ah, sure," thinking, *If only he knew.* I looked the other way, grinning. (We girls are SO bad.)

But I'm coming clean now. This afternoon, I started with some cookies at work. The cook was *not* impressed with me *at all* and he wanted no part of it whatsoever! But that's okay, he still loves me. He has been one of my biggest supporters from the very beginning. I still remember him telling me, "Drink that water!" when I found things really tough when starting.

Today, kids were having cheese sandwiches as a snack, so I took just one triangle of those. When he saw that, he got rid of the extras fast!

"Hey," I said.

"Nope! Not with me," he replied.

"Fine, then!"

(God love him, though.)

It's funny, but people are more scared than I am. I pretty much know what I can and can not handle, and I also know what I have to do in order to come out of it safe when times like these happen. Sometimes, that means hitting all the points, and then I'm okay. If I choose to ignore something I'm craving and thinking about, when I KNOW I can have it, it makes it tougher for the next few days. (If that makes any sense.) And then something that could have been a one-day screw up, can become a multiple-day one.

Today's attitude was: "You know what? It's my birthday! I have the right to do this on this day if I choose to. I have worked my butt off. One day won't hurt. So just let me enjoy it, will you?"

Having said that, once I got home I thought: *It has to be all or nothing. I have to get it all out of my system, every single thing out there that I crave, even on the odd occasion. I have to get it all out, done with, before a new day starts.*

So that's just what I did. I bought a cake (so had one more piece), I had some ice cream, a piece of apple pie (got that one tonight because last time I didn't), some chips, some chocolate, a little bit of pasta (couple of spoonfuls), some liquorice . . . (I think that's about it.) (I wish I'd had just one piece of pizza, but didn't have time.) Oh, and I had a Quarter Pounder and a small fries from McDonald's.

I think that covers it. Because I'm so near the end, I don't think it'll hurt me. Right now, my stomach feels bloated and heavy but that's all. I tried a bit of everything. I think I might need a few Tums tonight, and won't be going to bed for a while. I'll probably avoid the scale completely on Monday because I cannot face a bad number after being so excited to see 144. But in the meantime, I plan to have a tea that I have every night, to get me back in the groove and ready to start this two-month final phase fresh tomorrow.

(I hope my trainer doesn't give me attitude tomorrow.)

Friday, September 12, 2008

Technically . . .

Thought I'd tease my friends a little. (I'm so bad.)

I know the rule. I'm *not* supposed to show you guys *any* pictures until the end (about eight weeks or so), but . . . I thought I'd submit just one, a behind shot. Technically, you still can't see me.

I realize that not all of you are into this part of the transformation (muscle part), but please keep in mind that this is a *total* body transformation project, so Rob and I are trying to go beyond the weight loss thing that most people do these days.

I'm not trying to win a "sexy" contest right now. All I'm out to achieve is to get people talking while following my story. I hope that by being open like this, I'll help others to get inspired to change themselves, to take what you have now — no matter where you stand — and basically turn it around. As you can see, anyone can do this! Perhaps you may not want to go to this extent, but anyone can take control of his or her own life, and live a whole *different* life starting today!

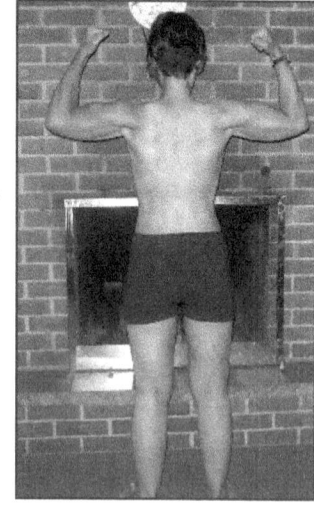

As you can see, things are still moving along quite nicely, changes are happening. Looking at this back shot, I was surprised: my arms are really changing big time. I couldn't help but ask: "Is that really me?"

This shows just how INCREDIBLE the human body can be! Going from the first two pictures where I was 275 pounds and *really* unhealthy (morbidly obese), then, in only ten months as of yesterday, you can see the most recent photo taken this morning at 144 pounds and really healthy! This is ALL NATURAL, remember? Pretty amazing!

November is fast approaching. Whatever will I look like?

Monday, September 15, 2008

After-Birthday Weekend

I visited my sister-in-law who has always been fairly petite. It was that time again, I needed a new wardrobe. We went through her stuff (some really nice stuff actually), and I came home with a garbage bag full of new pants. It helped me out big time because I'm going through sizes fairly quickly, so am trying to avoid purchasing much until the end. (When you can bet I'll be going on a massive shopping spree!)

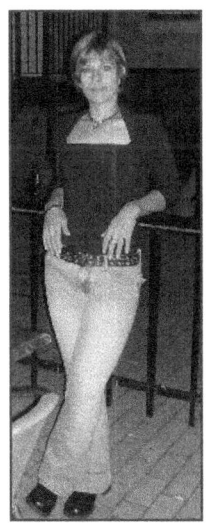

Whatever my weight might be, I've gone down in sizes once again! My weight has dropped. Sister-in-law gave me pants that were sizes 7 to 10. Nothing higher than that! I was very excited to see those numbers! *Wow!*

This was taken on our night out Saturday before I got into the wine.

Wednesday, September 17, 2008

Smooth Week!

I'm so excited to tackle the last weeks of this transformation, allowing myself to finish this off doing only my best. This week has been running a lot more smoothly (thank goodness). I think I've finally got down a routine for the kids, work, and workouts. That should make life easier.

I think it was something I had to get myself readjusted to, having the kids back in school, et cetera. Last year, just one child was in school, where this year, I have two in school and one in daycare, so it's been a little different. A lot more work, and a lot more running.

But that's okay. This is life for so many of us moms, so I shouldn't complain. They're only young once. I might as well enjoy them now while they still enjoy *me*. (I know there'll come a day when they might not want me around so much, or might even be a little embarrassed. I should count each day as a blessing! We might not have much, but we have each other, and that's the best thing one could ever ask for!)

Maybe everyone should keep this in mind when trying to accomplish something or to reach a goal: Always do whatever it takes to get to your goal while never losing sight of it! Some days might be tough, sometimes *really* tough. Things might come up that will leave you questioning your ability to continue. It's all about how badly you want it. If you want it that badly, somehow things just end up working out.

These last few days, I've been excited about getting through these next eight weeks! After my birthday weekend (drinking, forbidden foods), it was much easier than I thought it would be to get myself back on track.

I have to say something about going out eating and drinking. Since I don't do it that much anymore, or very rarely, I've noticed something.

The foods I ate — which, sadly, some people eat every single day — were very heavy on my stomach. You can definitely tell the difference! I even got pimples on my face, something I haven't had in quite a while. For the most part, my face has been clear throughout this transformation because of all the healthier foods, water, et cetera, but not after this past weekend!

It serves me right. When you eat garbage, that's what comes out, and that's basically what a lot of these foods are. Garbage.

Once you learn the right way of eating, and you've reprogrammed yourself, and you've gotten through the hardest part (which I believe is "adapting" to this whole new lifestyle, once you get to the phase where you're just "used to it"), the healthy way is what you like the most afterwards. The odd time, you might have a day of bingeing, but you now know the difference physically. You can tell, big time, what is good for you and what isn't just by how it affects you, inside and out. And it's such a nice feeling to know you can do that now. I don't think I could ever go back to the way I was and how I ate before, because of this.

ANYONE can achieve what I've achieved! You don't have to be a rocket scientist. We are each given a mind to think with, and to choose with, and the ability to do whatever it is we want in this life. We choose our own paths. It's all about choice and standing firm on any decision we make. Even though some of us have made mistakes, it's never too late to get back up, brush yourself off, and start fresh. That's the greatest thing about life. Every morning when the sun comes up, it's the start of a brand new day. That day can be whatever you want it to be.

Thursday, September 18, 2008

What Is Your Purpose in Life?

Today was one of those days when I found myself reflecting on what I've been through these past months, the journey through this whole thing, the ups and downs, and as I said to my trainer tonight, it's as if I were meant to finally tackle this obesity thing once and for all!

I remember an old friend, whom I haven't spoken to in years, who told me something that always stuck with me, an interesting way of looking at life, and the purpose of our lives here on earth. Now I'm not sure where you all stand religiously. I'm Roman Catholic, but at the same time I try to have an open mind concerning why we're all here. Let's face it, we really *don't* know. All we can go by is what we've been taught by our families, or the individual ideas we feel comfortable with. None of us can say we've experienced the other side and definitely know.

But the one thing I do believe, is that we're all here for "a special purpose." Some might not know what that purpose is, and might go through life trying to figure it out.

I remember what he said to me, how, to him, we have all been sent here to do something. A job, let's say, or a task, whatever that might be. It's almost like a test. Each life we live, we're given instructions before coming here. "Okay, this is your task. Let's see if you can conquer it or not." Every time we fail, we're brought back to try again. And again. And there are all these doors we must choose from, and paths . . . until we finally get it right. Once you get to that point, when you've finally passed the test, in your next life you'll be given a different task. Interesting? Kind of a neat way of thinking, I thought.

For some reason, regardless of my religious beliefs, that always stuck with me. Not sure why, but today I thought of that again. I also thought, *What if this was the task I had to tackle?* God knows it was a hard one! I've been big all my life, my weight started escalating in Grade 1 or 2. I knew nothing other than a life of being overweight. I suffered a lot through school. I was embarrassed to do many things the rest of the kids did. I would try to avoid gym time whenever I could. Obviously, I had to deal with the teasing. I was embarrassed to wear shorts. I was never asked out on dates. I would be the last one to be asked to dance at a high school dance.

As the years went on, I *could not* find it in me to change. I attempted many diets and workouts that would last a week at most . . . I'd come out feeling like I just couldn't do it. And I'd quit. A vicious circle.

And then finally, one day, one special day that I'll never forget, I made a decision. I believed in it. I knew in my heart I *was* going to do it this time, no matter what it took! And look at me today. After ten months, I can finally, finally say that I pretty much tackled it head on for the first time in my whole entire life at thirty-four years of age! I finally know what it's like to live a "normal" life, to not feel like an outsider, or not "good enough."

You can't imagine the feeling of personal accomplishment I'm experiencing unless you have at some time been in my shoes.

And so, I wonder, is this what I was supposed to do in my life?

Was this the challenge I was supposed to conquer? — Kind of a nice way to look at it, isn't it? — And helping others by writing about the whole thing, and letting the world in?

Look how a tiny idea that I called Rob about, grew so big. We have a blog that's viewed by hundreds of people a day, all over the world; we have our Facebook group; we have the *Ottawa Sun* newspaper following us; we have the Rogers 22 Daytime Show that we do; we have CNN watching us; and the book. It's INSANE, but at the same time, it's all flowed like it was meant to be. Everything's working out so perfectly in the time sense. I must say, however, I would *never* have imagined that so many people would be that interested in my story. I was hoping to touch a few people, but it grew!

I blogged it from day one. I kept going even when I found myself so busy some days I could barely think, but still, I fit in my blogs. Since starting, I felt this was a vital part of this journey for others, to actually live the life with me, instead of just through photographs. It's almost like a movie being played. For overweight people to read this and know they're not alone; to hear the emotions surrounding what it's like living the life and facing a challenge like mine; to hear the ups and downs of it all, will give them hope.

People (well, most people) are usually shy, and perhaps embarrassed to even think about doing what I did, open myself up about my life. But the one thing that worked for me was that all my life I was someone who would take chances. I've always done things that most people wouldn't even imagine trying. Sometimes they weren't the best things to do, but I always had the guts to do them, regardless.

In the beginning, people said: "Oh, how can you post those pictures?" "Everyone's watching and reading your personal stuff!" "What if you fail?" "I could never do that." . . . and on it went.

I knew this was something I had to do. If I were seriously going to finish this — and it was a risky chance, because I didn't really know if I could do it or not — I needed to blog it! It doesn't happen often that a person's world is one way, then all of a sudden, completely different. I mean, this story is as real as they come.

Anyway, it feels great to be this close to the end now. It really does. For once, to be given my chance at a different life, a different view on life. I've had a fighting energy inside me lately. I made it through this past week with no problems. I'll be ready on Monday to tackle the last seven weeks, hoping to reach my goal, while giving it all I've got! I'm almost there.

Please don't think it's easy to blog. It's not. You can't imagine how many times I go through it, rereading everything so it sounds the way I want it to. It takes a lot of time. But it's well worth it!

Monday's weigh-in will be the first after my birthday weekend. I'm nervous. But I can't hide forever. We'll find out just how much damage that caused. If any?

Monday, September 22, 2008

Crazy Morning!

What a crazy morning! I did my 6:00 a.m. cardio, then came home to bring the kids to the doctor, then went to the pharmacy to get their medication ... But when I came out of the pharmacy, the car wouldn't start. The battery was dead. I had to get a boost. Then over to our friends at Canadian Tire we all went. (Thanks, boys.) We had a new battery installed. Back home, lunch for the kids, I ate my grapefruit, and now I'm off to work.

I'll have to tackle my weight training after work today!

My weight: 143 pounds.

Saturday, September 27, 2008

No More Excuses. Just Do It

Phew! I made it through another work week. That means, if I can make it to Monday, it will then be six more weeks left. I can't believe it. I'm almost there! What a rush! It's like counting down to something REALLY BIG, like New Year's or something. Well ... then again ... It will be like New Year's to me.

178

I wonder if it's going to rain?

Before breaking the 200-pound mark — you might laugh at me, but — while doing my cardio, I thought: *When I break that 200-pound mark, I hope it rains outside. I hope it pours just to represent everything that I've been through until now, I hope it rains to wash away that life of being bigger than 200 pounds.* And you know what? That morning it *did* rain! I kid you not! The morning I weighed myself and it said 190 something, I was at the gym doing my cardio, and it rained!

I never told anyone about that. It might have been a coincidence and all, but I felt like the rain, as I watched it falling to the ground, was a huge weight lifting off me for the very first time! You have to remember that I was over 200 pounds for many, many years. Reaching that goal was a huge stepping stone for me!

Yes. I hope it rains again. I hope it pours. When that happens, it seems to represent all the hard work, the tears and sweat, and my crappy life before, and people laughing at me, and being embarrassed, and missing out with my kids — all those negative ways in which I chose to live because of stupidity, because I never took control of it. Ridiculous now that I look back. SO RIDICULOUS! Ridiculous that I allowed my body to first of all *get* that big, then to just accept it that way. Live that life. It might be tough to change, but to accept living a crappy life like that? Being sad all the time? Crying that no one will ever love me . . . and I DID IT TO MYSELF! We do it to ourselves! WE make that choice. Now, after only ten and a half months, I have a whole new life! Come on! We all can do it!

179

Yes, it's hard. Yes, it takes dedication and determination. Yes. You might have to let go of those shitty man-made foods we eat all the time. But SO WHAT? Our lives and our freedom are way more important than some cheap food we bought to stuff our faces with!

By the way, you'll still be able to have those crappy foods later, so it's not the end of the world, it's temporary. Rid yourself of them for now, as if they don't even exist. You must learn a new habit, one of control. That's all. Imagine being healthy, being confident, and learning how to enjoy healthier meals throughout the week, and on the weekend having a day to eat whatever you want to reward yourself. You go to the gym three times a week for forty minutes to maintain. That's it! What's so hard about that? The most difficult thing when you're obese or overweight, is getting to your personal ideal weight. Because everything you do counts: (a) You can do it in two to three years, going slowly, falling off the wagon and getting back on, by sometimes going to the gym, then missing for a few weeks; by saying "One day here or there won't hurt me if I eat this"; or (b) You can do it at a faster pace, by not giving in to bad things, by cutting out everyday foods, fast foods, foods that are high in fats and sodium, treats, sugar (all those foods that are bad for us and we all know what they are); by starting to work out at the gym, or at home if you have exercise equipment; and just by getting that body moving some way, some how. You just have to get it done.

I decided to pick "(b)" because I had wasted enough of my life. I wanted it done and over with. Once and for all!

I'm almost there. I've proven how a person can change, and it didn't take me much time. It wasn't some miracle drug I took. It was merely by wanting it badly enough, eating healthily, and working out five days a week. We all need to learn to stay focused when on a transformation journey, to stop allowing excuses to lead us astray. You need to get it done? *Get it done.* Start today!

When I started, I mentally prepared myself. I said: "No more! I don't care what happens, I'm going to do this!" I started looking at it as another job.

Most of us go to work every day. We have to be on time for work; there are always days we don't feel like going, or even getting ready to go, but we go. We know if we don't go, no money, so it's a must. Start looking at our bodies the same way: If we don't go, we won't have the healthy bodies we want and deserve!

Maybe by looking at it that way, when days come up that are hard, just think and say to yourself, "I hate going, but I have to." Get up and go! That's it. Once you're there, you'll see the hardest part was getting there. When you're about to work out, think: *The faster I start, the faster I'll be done.* And that's *exactly* what I used to say to myself. I kid you not. And it helped. Because I fully accepted that I needed to do this, that's it, that's all.

Remember! No excuses! You're the one who makes that final decision as to what sort of life you'll be leading, and what your body is going to be like in that mirror when you look back at yourself.

All I can say is, I feel *wonderful* and it was *well worth it!* So give it your best shot. Never give up!

Monday, September 29, 2008

A Great Reading to Start the Final Six Weeks

Today's weight: 139 pounds.

Total weight loss to date: 136 pounds.

Weight to drop by November 11: 14 pounds!

I have to say I was happy with the scale's reading this morning. It sets this week off on the right foot, makes me want to do really well! Now that I'm in another phase, the 130s, my main focus is to get out of them! No time to enjoy the victory of reaching the 130s.

After a talk with my trainer over the weekend, I mentioned how we have to average roughly 2 pounds per week to get to the 125-pound mark by November 11. His response: "Hard to do, but possible."

I won't even look at it that way. For me *it will be done!* My body cannot fail me now. Not when we are this close to the end.

For my workouts, I've started to mix up my cardio sessions: fifteen minutes on the bike, fifteen on the treadmill running, fifteen on the rowing machine. One reason I'm doing this is to make each exercise go by faster, and also because I think my body will do better if I mix things up a little.

Right now, I don't want my body getting used to *anything* that might make it slow down on me. This includes the cardio as well. I'm playing it up a bit to see what works best. I really like the way I feel after doing the combination, because the bike

focuses on my legs, and then the treadmill . . .
well, it's just plain tough to run. I feel the row
machine works everything from my arms to my
legs, so I think I picked a good combo.

I also have a gazelle from Tony Little that I use at
night sometimes for extra if I have the energy. I
really like that machine, and always have because
it doesn't put a lot of strain on your knees. Even
though I still have problems with one of my knees
for some reason (despite the fact I've come down
so drastically in weight), it's important for me not
to do anything to strain it. I can't afford to hurt my
body in any way, not now that we are on the
home stretch!

October 2008

Thursday, October 2, 2008

Challenging Last Few Days

Just got home, settled the kids with a snack, got a load of laundry in, and now munching on a few celery sticks as I try to write.

The last few days have been somewhat difficult. Wow. Not even sure how I got through them. Today, as I walked into my place of employment after my workout, the coworkers who were the first to greet me, said I looked drained.

I came into work dragging my feet, and my face was so blah (no expression), I felt as though I was pretty much "done," both mentally and physically. I felt like I'd been run over by something. Didn't help that today was Weight Training Leg Day (the routine that I find the most intense). I think it's all starting to catch up to me all of a sudden.

What my trainer and I have been tackling is pretty extreme. To actually do what we have done in such a short period of time, taking a body from morbidly obese to where it is now, in fewer than eleven months, is pretty insane. Obviously, there *will* be days where it'll hit me. All the changes I've gone through have been tough at times.

It has taken a lot out of me, mentally and physically. Now that I've been working on "other" projects, perhaps I have a little too much on my plate.

I'm at the stage where it's more of a *mental* game. I try to stay focused, but some days it's tempting to say "I'm done. This is it. I can't take any more of this seriousness."

Even when at the gym, I'm thinking *I'm almost there. Almost there.* These days, I find I have to remind myself of how far I've come, what my personal goal was from the beginning, and why it's so important that I give it my best shot right until the end.

Today when I was talking with Mike who works with me, I told him, "I don't know how much more I can handle." I took a deep breath. "I'm almost finished. Not sure I have any more strength in me to continue on at this level."

His response: "Rosy. I don't want to hear that from you. See this shoulder? It's *not* for you to cry on. You keep it going until you're finished. No quitters allowed. I won't hear it!"

"I know. I suppose I'll just drown myself and my thoughts in my water for now."

"There you go!" he said.

He says it like it is. That's probably why we get along so well. Talking to me like that, helps bring out the fighter in me. It's so easy, when things get tough, to start focusing on negative thoughts, and the idea of quitting. If you get too caught up in all that, it can cost you. At times, it'll take someone like Mike to flip it around!

He really knows how to talk to me to get me back to being focused on what means the most to me, and to get my mind away from negative thinking. He knows how badly I've wanted to reach this personal goal, and I guess for him, seeing that I've come this close, he would never support me if I chose to be a quitter now.

He has seen me every day since the beginning; he's watched me change as time passed, as I gradually became a healthier, more confident, and stronger person (inside and out). (Something I wasn't — at all — before starting this.) My life has completely done a 360-degree turn-around.

But even though I'm feeling drained, I also feel I need to do this. A while ago I said that I can't leave a story unfinished. Whether I make the 125-pound mark or not is not the big factor here anymore. The big factor is knowing that I gave it my all. That's the only thing that really matters to me right now.

No matter what, I'll come out of this a winner. And I also realize that no matter WHAT that scale reads on November 11, this part of our transformation project will be over! I'll be given a whole new life to enjoy. By my completing this, my friends, fellow bloggers, and ALL those people who have been following my story will, in turn, have their own hope back!

THIS is what this story *really* represents: giving people back the hope they perhaps lost along the way. This goes for whatever goal they might have. Whether it's weight related, or something on a completely different scale, it's all about going after what you want. Believe in yourself, and never underestimate what a human body and mind can do!

Well, I suppose this sums up my entry for tonight. I actually feel better now. I'm ready to finish off this week with a really good arm workout tomorrow, and I look forward to relaxing over the weekend (whenever possible). Then starting Monday, as we hit the last five weeks . . .

We're getting there! Soon.

Sunday, October 5, 2008

Comparing . . .

I guess my trainer wasn't joking when he said: "The end is going to really test your mental strength and will be the toughest time ever."

The end is definitely the hardest part! And I don't really believe it's the actual foods that make it that way. If I take a moment to reflect, I think it's more that you're relaxed, you can now see your goal so close by, you can almost touch it. You feel as though you might have time to waste now. You feel you can handle it. There are so many reasons like the ones I've just listed! But whether it be the next morning, or after a short period of time, once you stop stuffing your face because your stomach can't handle any more, you don't feel *any* better emotionally, no different than if it were your first cheat when you do screw up.

You still deal with that really crappy feeling. *That* stays the same. You always feel just as bad as you did when you cheated the very first time.

How do I feel after I eat bad stuff? I think it's important I talk about that for a moment to compare.

Let's compare . . .

For instance, when doing well, When I've had a great week, didn't cheat, had great workouts, I might find myself exhausted, yet feeling like I'm on top of the world! Nothing can bring me down. Nothing!

Other feelings I have:

great as a person
so fantastic
so strong
you can conquer anything
pretty
confident
positive
sociable
. . . smiling

When cheating, all of a sudden I don't feel happy anymore. I'm not sure if it's the actual foods which do that to you, all that junky man-made stuff, fried stuff, sweet stuff, whatever . . . Or is it mental?

But here are the changes in feelings:

I feel low as a person all of a sudden
I feel like the weakest person ever
I feel ugly
I feel paranoid, with thoughts racing through my
    mind such as *Are my legs getting puffy? Am I
    looking fat again?*
I feel defeated
I feel I've lost THE fight that a trainer trains so hard
    for
I feel I'm not so "high up" anymore
I can't believe I've screwed up all my hard work
    now!
Is my body going to change?
It was so natural the other night, what's going on
    inside now that reflects the outside?

What if people see what I did just now?
Am I going to start having to deal with cravings
    again?
Am I going to have to deal with getting my
    control back?
Why did I even do that?

Just look at the emotional differences we deal
with as an after-effect of cheating. I don't think it's
the foods that screw you up later, that make the
"cheat" turn into disaster. I think it's all the
negative and *bad* feelings that take over our minds
and bodies. Then we feel like failures, like we
can't do it, and we give up.

Makes a kind of sense, doesn't it? It's amazing
that our mind is so powerful and can do that. If
we always focus on how we lost one night, how
we gave in, then that's probably the reason why
most people end up not finishing what they set
out to do.

But just like admitting your weight in the
beginning, I think it's important to come clean
when you screw up. If I chose to hide it, it would
only give me an excuse to make a cheat become a
bad habit again.

That's one thing I don't want: an excuse to go back
to being unhealthy again! I have to deal with what
I've done, and as the owner at Free Form Fitness
says: "Get up. And start again!"

Meantime, no matter what, I feel that I have to be
completely honest as I go through this, so others
might understand how tough it can be. How
tough it was as a weak person in the beginning,
and ALSO how tough it is for a strong one. It's

always tough! Now I'm starting to think it's something that must be tough on *everyone*. Not only you and me, the ones fighting a weight problem, but people in general.

Tuesday, October 7, 2008

Monkey See, Monkey Do
<u>Another Milestone to Talk About.</u>
What an interesting day at the gym it was! Sometimes, when I least expect it, my body will surprise even me!

About three weeks ago, I was at Free Form Fitness with the owner, Chelsea, and together we tried to have me do a chin up. No way! That was not going to happen!

Although I really tried, I never realized how tough doing a chin up was. It might look easy (not to mention, make someone look physically strong, especially if a woman does it), but *man*, I could only get my body half way up to the bar, if that.

Today? Different story altogether!

I tried it again. To my surprise, I am pleased to say: Up, up I went like a monkey swinging in his glory! Okay. Maybe not swinging, but I managed to lift my body, and get my chin right up and even over the actual bar! *Wow!* I thought! *This is great!* It was the best feeling in the world.

Couldn't do any more, of course, but the fact that I was able to do even *one*, shows that no matter what that scale might read, I know for a fact I must be getting down in weight (or leaner), and that my arm strength must be building at a rapid pace now.

Saturday, October 11, 2008

One Mind, One Focus, One Goal: To Make It!

Funny thing. Not sure if you've ever noticed, but when you're in a slump or in a bad mood, it seems like everyone around you is, too.

But this week, because I was in a good mood, it just seemed like people were smiling more as they passed on the street, or in the stores. You bring your positive energy to work and it gets passed on to your coworkers, you find yourself saying good morning to everyone, and really meaning it, and there's a certain positive energy in the air! It's nice when this happens. If only we knew how to keep that going, the world would be a much happier place (with fewer grumps).

Monday, October 13, 2008

Happy Thanksgiving to All

I'm pretty sure everyone by this time is getting that big turkey stuffed and ready to go. Thank goodness I'm not cooking this year, I won't have to put myself through all those great smells until later tonight when I go to my brother's house.

Even though it's Thanksgiving, you know me, I'm getting ready for the gym. With only four weeks left — twenty-nine days, to be exact — I'm in a race with the clock.

Today's weight wasn't the best. Was disappointed in the reading. I was only able to hit 140 pounds.

Knowing my body, next week is when the big plunge will come. This tends to happen by the second week afterwards. (This is what I'm hoping for, at least.)

Later — Thanksgiving Dinner

Dinner went well tonight. It was tough, especially when I had to give up tasting the fresh pumpkin pie, apple pie, apple crumble pie, chocolate ice cream, chocolate cookies, whipped cream . . . *Wow!* That's all I can say.

It was tough — you know how I love and crave my sweets the most — but I was mentally prepared for it. I just reminded my family, twenty-nine days, and after that, when a special occasion comes up, I, too, will be able to enjoy some of those yummy delicious treats!

I think they felt a little bad. After all, my sister-in-law had a great variety this year to display and choose from. I just bent over and enjoyed the smell of everything. Anyway, no more talking about that tonight, I need to go to bed and not think twice about it. I need, instead, to think about getting up in the morning for a forty-five-minute cardio session. Something much more important!

Sunday, October 19, 2008

Monday Weigh-In

My life has changed so much, I can't even begin to say how, it's impossible to describe. However, even today, at the weight I am, I still find myself thinking thoughts (when seeing my reflection) that I'm not as slim as some people say I am. It's really strange.

Perhaps it's because, when you've been obese, or overweight, all your life, the only thing you really ever knew was: "I need to lose weight," not the opposite. This is something I'll have to work on later. Really, with the little amount of weight that I have left to lose, it won't make a huge difference in my appearance — there won't BE much left of me! I suppose it's something else I'll have to work on, like the maintenance.

This whole thing has moved so fast for me that I haven't had time to adjust, even to the different parts of my life that have changed. It's been such a mentally and physically crazy time, that there was really never any time to look at and see and understand what I've tackled and accomplished. It moved too fast.

People who see my photos, and who've heard my story, are shocked at the rapid changes. I'm left there testifying: "Yes. I *did* do it naturally by working out and eating properly."

The body is an amazing thing. I feel blessed that I was able to take this journey because, when I reflect on it, through watching every change, I realized I'd never seen anything like it in my life.

Sunday, October 26, 2008

Sometimes the Stars Line Up Everything for You

Meet Hedley, My Favourite Canadian Band!

Boy! Do I have a story for you today! Go grab a coffee or a tea or whatever and make sure you have time because this story is a long one — but a funny, exciting, and unbelievable one that will have you chuckling: "The Life of Rosy and the Stuff I Get Myself Into."

As I mentioned before, one of my all-time favourite Canadian groups is Hedley. Not sure if you've ever heard their music, but it's their music that in the beginning got me through a lot of tough times. A lot of their songs have a kick-butt attitude, a don't-care attitude, so pretty much always got me pumped to get through the days. I really like them.

They were in town yesterday for a book signing. They just had their book released, *Fan Lowdown*, and their most recent CD, *Famous Last Words*. (Get out and buy one if you get a chance!)

My friend, Sonia, and I decided we were attending the book signing at Chapters on Rideau Street. We were sad that we couldn't get any tickets for the sold-out general admission , even though I didn't want any actual "seats" — I like to get in there where all the energy is!

So picture this like a movie playing, here goes:

So Sonia and I are in the lineup to meet our favourite band. We are trying to get through the wait-time of four hours before they arrive. (We figured we should get there early because there's a limited number of wrist bands given out and we did *not* want to miss out on *that* event since we *would* be missing the concert afterwards.)

I had brought my scrapbook with me, hoping that somehow I might be able to use that to convince the group to give their Biggest Fan some tickets for the show. It was a chance I was taking, but I was up for the challenge.

Losing weight and coming as far as I have in this transformation project, has returned my confidence. I've always had guts (to publicize this whole transformation story from beginning to end just shows what kind of guts I have). But talk about having to go above and beyond my usual! I knew what I wanted, and I was ready to go for it. It was my turn to shine!

We were only seven people away from the front of the line when the Hedley group arrived.

I told Sonia: "No. We need to go to the back!"

"What?" She couldn't believe what she was hearing, but my gut instincts said "back."

I knew if we went to the back of the line, we'd probably be given more time to talk, I wouldn't feel so rushed — nor would the group — because there'd be no one behind us. It just made sense.

So we'd rushed to Chapters for nothing! But like I said, the stars were lining up for me at this point. Everything happens for a reason. Right?

Here we are. It's our turn. I walk right up, looking confident, thinking positive thoughts like: *You're bigger than they are. You're bigger than they are. You can do this, Rosy.*

My friend knows, if anyone can do this it, I can. She's an even bigger fan of Hedley than I am, so she's hoping and praying I can pull this off. (I'm left with the pressure of making it happen.)

I start off by placing my scrapbook, with all the newspaper clippings, my month-to-month photos, et cetera, on the table in front of lead singer, Jacob Hoggard. Looking back, I didn't realize I was actually in Jacob's face, so close to him, bent over, with my face in his, and I'm giving him the summary as quickly as I can, but in a serious way:

"Listen, Jake. Last year around this time, I had one mission. And that mission was to lose 150 pounds in one year."

Sonia says: "Yeah. She weighed 275 pounds!"

I'm thinking: *Shut up, Sonia!*

Jake, surprised, says: "Oh, really?"

"I'm only two weeks away from my goal and at your last concert I purchased a shirt that was a size small. It didn't fit me at all, but it helped inspire me to really kick ass to do this and basically I promised myself the next time you boys would be in town, I'd be wearing it to show you."

I zipped open and removed my leather jacket, so they could see that I was wearing the shirt, and how great it looked. (I was even able to flex for them!)

It was hilarious!

They seemed proud, happy, and shocked all at once. I'm sure they've heard many stories, but mine is definitely one they won't forget, I doubt if anyone ever told them a story like *that* before.

They all gave me hugs and stuff. Really nice, and asked if I'd be attending the concert that night.

Here goes my magic.

"Actually," I said. "Come to think about it, I really wanted to because we've been to every concert, and we tried to get floor seats, but there were none left, so sadly, no." I tried to smile and look sad at the same time. "I'm hoping you can help us out and get us some."

Next thing you know, some guy walks up. "Okay," he says. "What's your name and how many you want?"

"Really?" Thinking, *It was that easy?*

So I just said a number. "Five." I don't know why. And here I was, *Wow. We got backstage! Oh. My. Gawd.* My eyes were huge, popping out of their sockets!

I hugged everybody. "Thank you. Thank you. Thank you." I was so excited.

Back at the car, Sonia and I were pumped. "It worked! It worked! We are going tonight! And we are going backstage!" (This is what we thought, right?)

So we rushed to a store first to pick up a cake to bring along. We had them write something on it. (That's the Italian in me. You can't show up somewhere and not bring anything. Right?)

We were rushing to get there, wanting to be early enough to hang out with the band a bit before the show, so we only had time to go back to my place, freshen up the makeup, change my belt, and off we went.

The funny thing is, when we drove up — again, talk about everything just lining up perfectly —

who happens to walk by us? Who had parked only a few cars over? The drummer, Chris Crippin, and his wife.

Perfect! I thought. "Come on, Sonia! Let's go!"

Picture this: Me with my umbrella and my book, and the banner we'd brought. Sonia with this huge cake, running a few feet behind me. It's raining. And we notice that Chris is going into a back entrance where the public doesn't go.

"Who cares. Let's go," I told Sonia.

She's more nervous than I am. "I don't know, Rosy. Should we be doing this?"

"Never mind," I said.

So we get to the door and the security guard asks: "Are you with them?"

"Yes. See? We have the cake." (We were meant to buy that cake!)

"Okay. Go ahead then."

I can't believe I'm doing this, I think.

The security guard even helps me with the door because my umbrella is getting stuck in it. (I was on such a high, I forgot to close it.) I said — so politely — "Oh. Thank you."

"No problem. It's the least I can do." He laughs. "Go have fun."

So here we are following them. It's dark and

tunnel-ish. Then some other guy asks if we're with them.

"Oh, yeah. Ask Chris." So I yell out to the drummer who's not too far ahead, but still hasn't noticed us trailing him: "Hey, Chris!"

He turns around, see me and says: "Yeah. Yeah. They're fine."

Chris was in such a rush himself, that he probably didn't even know how I got there, or why, but he didn't really care. It was all working out as planned.

We followed them downstairs to the band's eating area. The tables were set up buffet style.

Chris says: "Oh. Just set the cake on the table there."

"Okay. Sure," I said.

Sonia and I stand there gawping at each other like we can't believe it. (She's been going along with whatever I've been doing.)

There were a few "important people" in the room, so I decided I'd better introduce myself, make myself look important as well. So I'm going around saying: "Hi. I'm Rosy." I'm shaking their hands. They're responding warmly, telling me their names, and shaking mine back. (Sonia's behind me doing the same thing. This is really funny because she's more the nervous type and I'm imagining how nervous she must have been about this whole situation!)

Then the guy who had originally marked my name on that piece of paper at Chapters came up to us. He looked at me a little oddly, but at that point, with all the chaos going on around, no one asked questions, like how we were even *in* there to begin with. Probably, everyone had a million other things on their mind, and weren't thinking about it.

The guy looked at me and said, "Well. You'll have to take your stuff into the change room for the Meet and Greet. The guys will be there soon to take pictures, and sign."

"Sure," I said. "No problem." So we grabbed our stuff and went into the other room.

Sonia and I were the first ones in there. Can you believe that? We placed our banner on the table in the middle of the room, along with the cake, and my scrapbook I wanted them to sign. (I HAD to get a picture of it all to prove what I did!)

Suddenly, about twelve people walk in (some kids with their mothers), plus Security. We had no idea who these people were, but I had my ears and eyes open, taking it all in, "going with the flow."

Some other event guy walks in with a walkie-talkie and says they'll be in in a few minutes, and says we should line up shoulder to shoulder. (I was thinking *Last year again, we're back in jail, but it's okay. Go along, Rosy.*)

Then he started going around the room asking everyone (conversationally, I suppose) how they got in there and who they knew. I realized that the few people in there were people who "knew"

someone, either a business person or someone
with connections. Then there was me. And Sonia.
Just standing there. When he got to us, all he said
was: "I suppose you two are just super fans?"

Smiling, I responded, "Uh. Yeah. That's right."

Next thing I know, the group walks in. (Good
timing, man!) My heart is pounding. I'm thinking:
*Any time now, we are going to be kicked right out of
here.* (I'm realizing that Sonia is probably freaking
out even more than I am because she's already so
nervous, but I had no time to think about Sonia, I
had to keep going along and get through it, and
keep the smile going. At this point, I'm thinking
that the only thing saving my butt is my smile.)

So when the boys got to us, they looked sort of
surprised, but yet again, there was so much going
on they didn't question us. "So," they said,
smiling. "Nice to see you girls again."

We got more hugs and had all our stuff signed.
We took a picture with the cake. All nice, nice,
laughing. I chatted with them a bit, me my joking
self as if I've known them forever and they were
my best friends. Jake, the lead singer, made a
comment like, ". . . oh why don't you eat some
cake with us?" . . . laughing. I said " . . . don't
tempt me, I'll eat the whole thing " . . . laughing
back. (If only he knew how serious I was!)

After that, we were all directed to follow another
security guard because the show was about to
start. We picked up our stuff, leaving the cake for
them, and walked along with the group of other
"special" people that were allowed to be there —
unlike the "sneaks" that Sonia and I were.

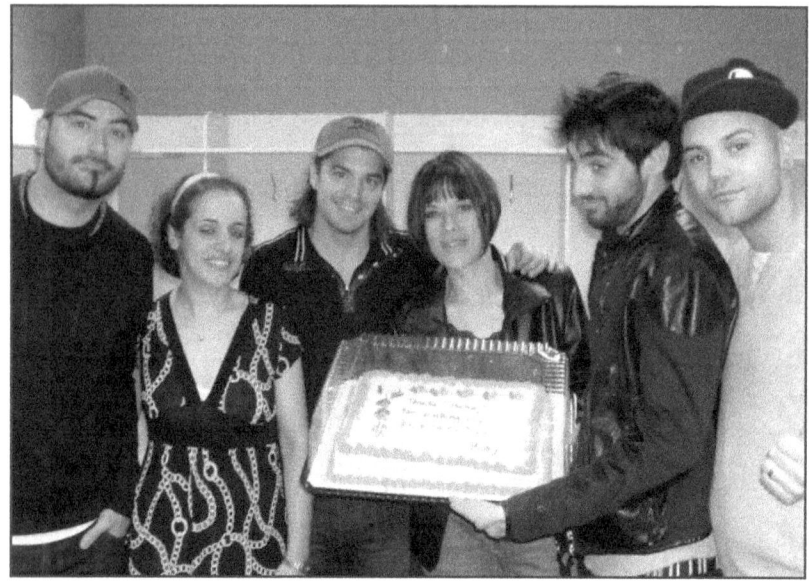

Left to right are Tommy Macdonald, Sonia, Chris Crippin, Me, Jacob Hoggard, and Dave Rosin.

Well . . . When we got to the end of our walk, we had to present our "tickets." *Oh, gawd. How am I going to get out of this one?*

So when it was our turn, I just said "Well. We never *got* any tickets!"

"What do you mean?" the guy says.

"I dunno. That promotional guy just put our names on the list at Chapters, so we didn't pick up any tickets."

"Oh."

(I was freaking out.)

"Well. Okay then. Your name must be at the box

office. Just go up there and they'll give you your tickets for the show."

Phew.

Off we go to the box office. "Well. I guess this is it," I say to Sonia. "I suppose there's no more backstage. But, hey! We got to experience something a lot of people don't. We should be happy."

But it doesn't stop there . . .

When getting our tickets at the box office, I notice they gave us five seats in the upper level. Upper level? *Oh, no. Sonia is afraid of heights. What am I going to do?*

So the walkie-talkie guy comes along, and I decide to ask him.

Casually, I say: "Oh. They must have made a mistake. I told them at Chapters today, that we wanted floor seats because my friend here is

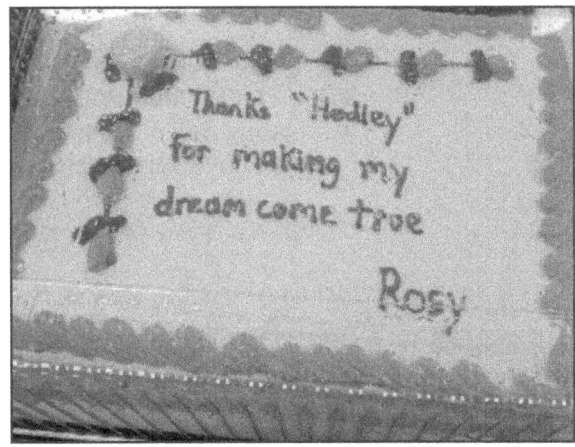

afraid of heights and we can't be sitting that high."

Sonia puts in her two cents worth, too: "Yeah," she says. "I get heart palpitations."

I'm trying not to bust up laughing.

The guy says, "Well you know, you really should be happy with getting what you got. Other people would see it as getting something free. You should be grateful."

"Oh. We are. But I don't know what to do now."

"The only thing you can do is go back to the box office people and ask them. I *highly* doubt they'll change them because the floor is sold out. Has been for months. But . . . doesn't hurt to ask."

I told Sonia, "Look, I'll try. But I don't know about this one. If not, we either take the seats given or go home."

Back to the guy at the box office, me with my winning smile. "Hi there." (Smiling.) "Sorry to bother you . . ." And I start. "I just noticed that these seats are high and honestly my friend has an issue with heights here . . . so I was wondering if there's any way possible we could get floor seats. I would really appreciate it so much."

"Well. Who issued you these seats anyway?"

"Oh. I don't know his name. He's just someone who takes care of promotions for the group. He put us on the list today when the group was at Chapters signing their book."

"Hmm. Let's see." (He's thinking.) "Okay."

Just like that he said okay! I couldn't believe our luck!

In our hands are general admission tickets! Something we wanted from the beginning and we got so much more! We got to meet the group. We got to hang with them — what an awesome experience! I really believe it was meant to be.

I remember looking around the room at the thousands of people there, while the lights were on them, and I knew that this was what it's all about! I had to write about this. I could NEVER have pulled this off if I was who I was last November. My confidence wouldn't have been strong enough. When you feel confident, and believe in yourself, and believe in good things, it pours out. People see it and feel it. It happens! Things happen for you!

Everything last night was all about timing. It was all meant to be! From going to the back of the line at Chapters, to arriving at the concert at the same time as the drummer, to getting backstage, to the Meet and Greet, to the floor tickets . . . What are the chances of that? Something I would dream about, but never thought I'd experience.

Driving home, Sonia and I laughed and laughed. We could not believe the night we'd had. We honestly thought that taking our names at Chapters meant we were going backstage, when the reality was they were only going to provide us with tickets. But somehow we managed to do a lot more than that.

It's a night I'll never forget. Perhaps it's one of Life's ways of giving back to me. I don't know. But, hey! What a great and memorable time!

And the Hedley band were fantastic! They were genuinely happy about what I had done, and really supportive. I told them I was going to write about this in my book.

I plan to send them a signed copy of the book: *My* signature this time, instead of the other way around!

Friday, October 31, 2008

Twelve Days Left. Time for Reflection

Like I said before, I'll NEVER forget where I came from, and where I once was. How can I? I lived it for much of my life. No matter how great the shape I'm in today, or how people who never knew me back then see me today, that old Rosy will always be a part of me.

I'm sure the people who see me in the gym, those who don't know my story, probably think I've always trained like this. If they only knew! But, boy, did I ever work my butt off to get to where I am. Nothing comes easy. Nothing is handed to us. We have to fight for what we want. There's no reason to cry and feel sorry for ourselves, because we choose what we eat, and what we do. If you want to change, DO IT!

Now that my personal transformation project is coming to an end soon, I'm feeling weird about it. I'm thinking to myself, *Did I make a difference in someone else's life by taking them through this journey with me? Did I inspire anyone to make a change like I did? Was I able to affect people like I wanted to?*

I'm not going to weigh myself now until the end. Whatever that scale reads, we'll let it read. I'm going to keep going to the gym every day until then, giving my workouts all I've got, I'm going to eat exactly what I'm supposed to be eating, and that's the best I can do.

But no matter what that scale reads, I'm so happy right now, I couldn't *be* any happier. Even if I can't make that goal, physically, of being 125 pounds exactly, I'm pretty sure my trainer and I have proved the point. No matter who you are, you can accomplish whatever you want in life! So what if I'm only 5 pounds away from 125? Or 10 pounds away? I have kicked some serious ass, and I'm now living the life I should have been living a long time ago!

That's another thing on my mind. Would I actually disappoint people if I didn't make that number? Would they look at me as a failure? Most close friends I've discussed this with tend to say "No way! Look how far you've come, Rosy!" But I wonder.

Perhaps if I look deeper into the question, it's myself I might feel I've disappointed, because it was MY personal goal.

November 2008

Saturday, November 1, 2008

Rosy Has Gone into Hiding

. . . thinking this is the best way to keep focused on the end.

This morning, I was able to get in another cardio and weight-training session. Tomorrow, I plan to visit the YMCA to get in one more "just cardio" session as an extra.

I've decided that for the remaining eleven days, I will go to the gym every single day. No breaks.

I have also decided *not* to go out, or see any friends, and to even keep talking with them to a minimum. This includes my trainer.

In order to keep focused on getting to the end now, I need to let go of any stresses, or anything that might sidetrack me.

This last part is all up to me. The last numbers I read were 134 pounds. Those are the only numbers I will be seeing until the final on November 11!

I want to take a moment right now to thank my trainer, Rob Lagana, for all he has done for me. He is, and always will be, my angel who came to save me. He has taught me so much. The patience and support, and basic respect for me as a person throughout this journey, was very important to me, something I truly needed. I will never forget.

I believe we met up once again in this life for many reasons. I know I needed *him*. And I think I was the person *he* needed to prove that from his fourteen years of studying in this field, his theory on this weight loss and bodybuilding thing really works. His theory that food and exercise go hand in hand BIG TIME is valid. If you can stay on track mentally, and follow what he says, ANYONE can change for the better, and we aren't just talking little changes, but dramatic ones.

My biggest hope is that I have made him proud. He believed in me from the beginning. He probably believed in me more than I believed in myself at times. When there were harder days, days when I felt like giving in, all I had to do was think about him, and he would be my strength.

I will never forget the first time, and I know I said this before, but, when he came to assess me, and I had to weigh myself and take my measurements for the very first time in front of him, I was so embarrassed and ashamed. But, honestly, he looked at me with the same respect *that* day as he does today.

That's Rob for you.

Scruff, I think we have come a long way. At the time, I might have been the heaviest in weight that you had to work with, but you didn't seem worried at all. I think I was more worried than you were.

But now it's time for *me* to fly, to finish this journey alone. I just need to say that no matter what that scale reads on November 11, I'm so happy either way! I believe this is the most important thing. I cannot be any happier than I am right now, nor can I be in any better shape than I'm in today.

This has been such a journey, so many ups and downs, so much deep inner-soul searching, being challenged and tested constantly, then finally being able to find myself and who I really am. Somewhere, underneath all that fat I once carried, was a pretty tough chick, if I must say so myself. And you know what's great? We *all* have that toughness inside. You just need to find it, that's all. And once you do, never let it go.

Sometimes, I find myself tearing up because I have this whole new life now. No more being embarrassed. No more socks to cut because they won't fit around my ankles. No more saying to myself all the time: "I have to lose weight." No more being out of breath, no more Rosy coming last, no more names called out to me like in grade school. No more teasing, no more missing out with my kids. No more feeling ugly and unattractive.

I have so much to look forward to now. And you can *bet* I'll never go back to what I was before. No way. Too much hard work to get to this point. Remember, nothing comes free in life. You want something, you have to go and get it! You can cry and be sad and feel upset and sorry for yourself, but meanwhile, time just ticks away. The more you let it go, and not take control, the more you are cheating yourself. If you are overweight or obese — whatever — the bottom line is (whether you choose to admit to it or not): we are the ones to blame. We really do it to ourselves. It's up to us to take control and change it. It's about making a choice to live healthier and to stick to it no matter how hard it may get at times. It's all about remembering why you chose to start living better, and holding on to that.

I have a dinner on the 14th where I'll be seeing all my friends once again. We'll celebrate the end of this really strict and crazy time period of my life. And just as I find myself crying now while writing, I know I'm going to break down that day.

Sometimes, you can't help but break down if you've dealt with a lot mentally. There were many emotions running through my mind during it all, all the stresses of trying to keep everything going, along with the everyday pressures of my other life.

But when the time comes and I finally see my trainer, my friends, coworkers, and family sitting around the room together, as a big family, and I'm able to look at them all and say I did it. It's done. It will be the first time I'll be letting go of all those feelings and thoughts, and pressures. I'll finally be able to live my life freely in a whole different way.

It's been a tough and challenging twelve months. Really, really tough! I can picture the different parts of this transformation from beginning to end like a movie playing in my mind.

All my life I've said "I have to lose weight," "I have to lose weight." And every single time I tried, I would fail. That's all I knew: failure. But today I can stand proud and say I fucking did it! I stared it in the face, like my worst enemy, and I beat it! This time I beat it! I fought it right to the end!

(My hormones must be all out of whack right now. I'm tearing up like a baby.)

All I know is I have to do what I have to do in the next eleven days. Give it all I've got. Eat right and exercise to the max. Finish this off!

Monday, November 10, 2008

Twelve-Month Anniversary Pictures. The Wait is Over!

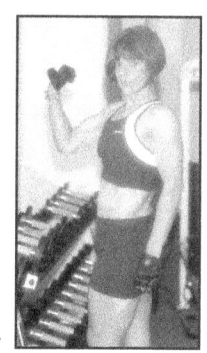

I decided to post my brand new twelve-month photos early. It's been a long wait for some of you, and now, they are here and released. Hope you enjoy them.

But first: weight.

As of this morning at the doctor's office, the scale read 132 pounds. I tried, but it's no biggie. The pictures are much more impressive, I think, and I can still hit 125 pounds in the next few weeks if I decide to go that route.

PHOTOS BY GORDON CHAN

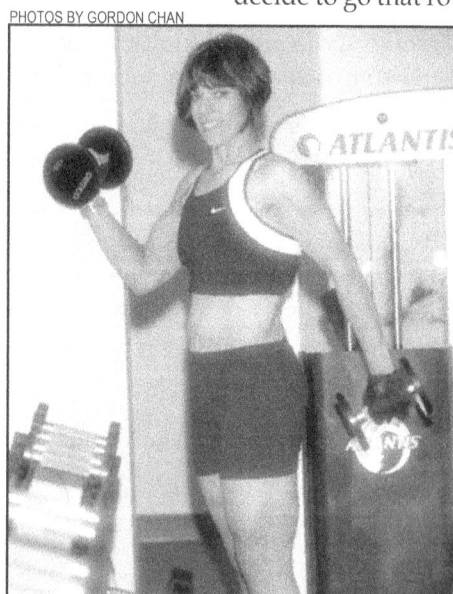

So . . .

I have officially lost 143 pounds in only twelve months. I was only 7 pounds shy of my original goal of 150 pounds, but incorporating the weight training has made that mark a little bit difficult to get to. But I suppose it still IS impressive when you realize that I did it in such a short period of time, all natural, no surgeries or quick fix pills . . . or starving myself. I can walk away happy! I think what my

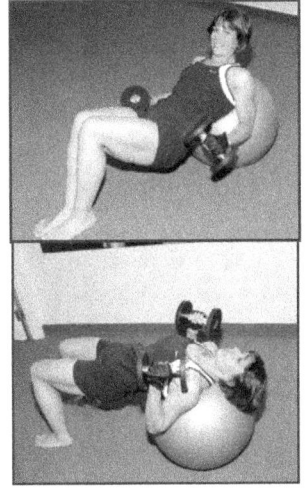

trainer and I set out to prove has been done. I hope I've set an example for all. Remember, we are much stronger than what we give ourselves credit for!

If *I* could physically change so drastically in only twelve months, it shows what we as humans can do once our minds are set! It's all mental. That's all it is.

I just want to say again, that this past year has been a tremendous mental and physical challenge, but I'm here, standing tall and proud. I beat the odds that were stacked high against me: I defeated my worst enemy — obesity — forever.

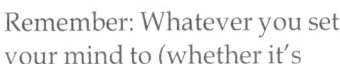

Remember: Whatever you set your mind to (whether it's weight related or not), you can have in this life. You have to want it badly enough, and you have to just go for it!

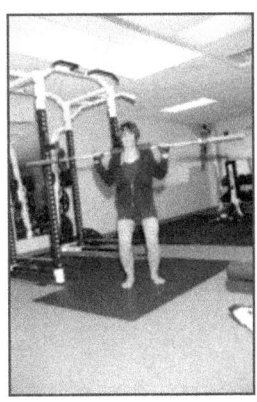

I love you all very much, and will never forget the support I received from all of you, and the kind words of encouragement. This is what kept me going each and every day.

PHOTOS BY GORDON CHAN

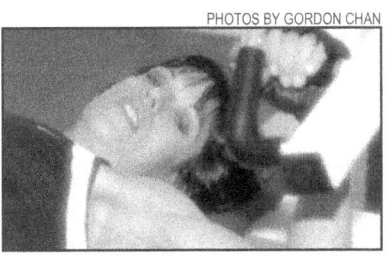

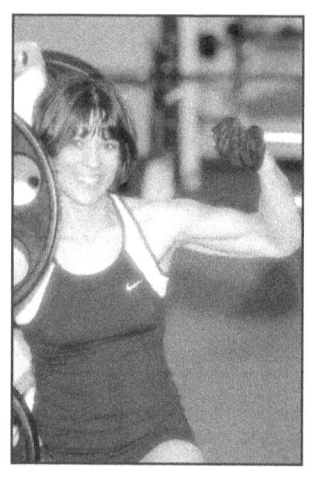

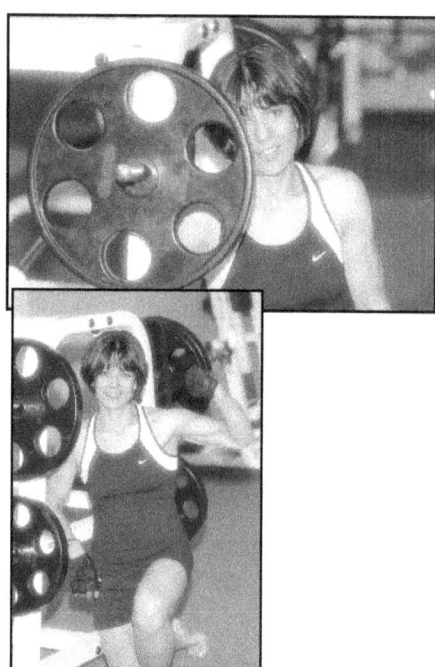

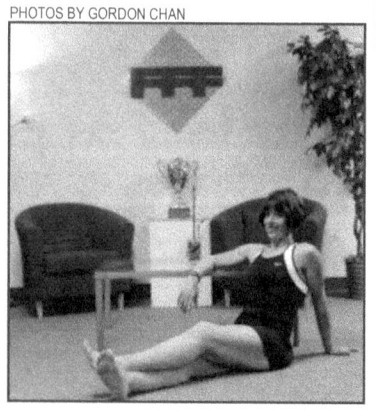

PHOTOS BY GORDON CHAN

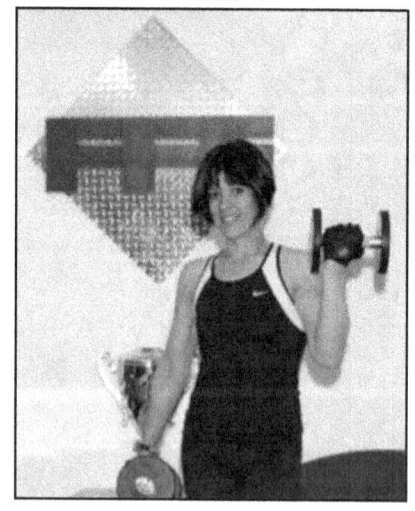

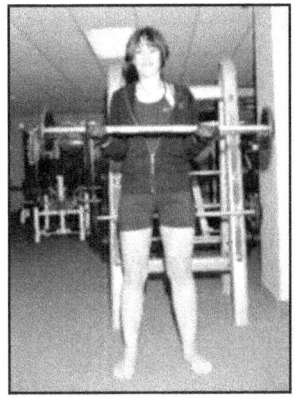

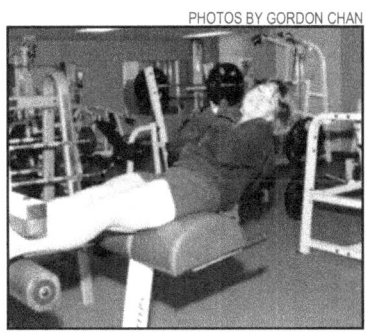

PHOTOS BY GORDON CHAN

Sunday, November 23, 2008

Always Keep Looking Ahead

As the tears fell down her face, her father looked at her and said ,while pointing to the tears, "What are they? Why do you allow them to fall? You need to stand up and wipe them away because things will only get better."

I wanted to write this morning because earlier on, my "emotional" state was not the greatest. It really had nothing to do with this transformation. I had a surprise visit from my dad.

During a phone call earlier, he had heard in my voice that I was upset about a few things I've been dealing with, so being the strongest man I've ever known, he came over to see me. (I'm blessed even to be able to call him my dad.)

Despite what people might think, this past year has been really tough at times, more than I've been letting on. I didn't talk about my "other issues," so people might have assumed I "have it made," that things are just handed to me, that I must have such an easy life.

Because I concentrated on talking mostly about areas regarding this project, everyone automatically thinks to themselves that things must be easy for her in other areas of her life, or she must not have much else she deals with. The truth of the matter is, just like many of you, I, too, have had some hard times this year. (Still dealing with them.) I'm trying to keep myself strong and focused, keep my hopes up that things can only get better.

I'm not sure why I wanted to post my dad's words from this morning's visit. Maybe those words can be applied to many things, including when we're trying to fight the obesity battle, a battle many of us are in. It takes everything you've got to succeed at some things. Sometimes it breaks you, but you need to find it in you to keep moving ahead, knowing that eventually, it'll have been worth it.

It takes a lot out of you to fight, to never give up, especially during those times when Life throws stuff at you, perhaps trying to throw you off.

Challenging ourselves with something we've always found difficult in our lives is probably one of the most beneficial, but yet most difficult, things we can do. For me, it was to change, to become a better, stronger person, physically.

We should be proud of *any* step we take toward making our lives better. The mere fact that you try makes you that much stronger than someone who hasn't tried.

I really look up to my dad. Like so many fathers, he was one who would do anything for his kids. Even though we're all grown up now, and living our own lives, he looks at us with such pride, and is still there to give a helping hand (or, like this morning, rich words of wisdom). Through the years, I've learned a lot from my dad, and I believe this is what has helped me become who I am today.

He's been through so much himself during his life, and no matter what hardships he may have had during that time, you'd never see a tear fall. Never! He is such a proud man. This book Rob and I are putting together, will be dedicated to my dad.

Even if no one were to buy this book, I'd be so happy to give him my first copy, and to say "I did it, Dad!" He is someone we could all strive to be like. Even though I might break at times, and show emotion, the bottom line is, I must have gotten that fighting spirit from him.

He is probably the reason why I'm even here, writing so openly to strangers. The guts I have to do things where I put myself out there, and to be so open and honest, stems from having such a strong father figure in my life. I took a chance going public with this whole thing. I could have failed. I could have been laughed at, but I did it to help other people, hoping that by reading my story others in the same spot might be helped.

I'm sure there are many, many people wondering how long I'll keep this weight off. Some are just waiting for me to put every single pound back on.

221

All I can say to that is, I'm taking it one day at a time. I know I don't EVER want to go back to where I once was, but like everything else, there are never any guarantees. But what I do know is, the freedom I've already had a chance to experience for the first time in my life, has been such a blessing, why would I want that taken from me, from my family — mostly from my kids? Is indulging in foods which ruin us more important than freedom? I don't think so. Will I have these foods from time to time, or maybe go on a week's binge? Probably. But this time, I know how to get back on before it gets out of control.

You'd better believe I will do everything in my power to stay straight, to always remember how far I've come, and how hard I worked to get here.

Ciao!

.

www.ingramcontent.com/pod-product-compliance
Lightning Source LLC
Chambersburg PA
CBHW060456290526
45791CB00001B/140